BMA

'Witty and elegantly written accounts of his medical practice'
The British Medical Journal

'The GP sitting in their consulting room never really knows what the next patient will bring. Launer, in his masterful collection of essays, recreates this element of surprise for the reader, illuminating the richness of the medical encounter. A gem, for doctors and patients, alike'

Dr. Caroline Elton, author of
Also Human: The Inner Lives of Doctors

'Witty and wise. Shows how important it is that doctors are allowed to be human' **Kit Wharton, author of** *Emergency Admissions: Memoirs of an Ambulance Driver*

'The nature and meaning of reflective practice by doctors is currently being hotly debated. Launer's entertaining read is also a timely and salutary reminder of the value of reflection' **Neena Modi, Professor of Neonatal Medicine, Imperial College London**

'These short, crystalline and deceptively simple essays go to the heart of what it is to be a doctor – and a patient. Launer addresses difficult issues with characteristic wisdom, honesty, humanity and wit. His insights are profound and will resonate with every clinician and with anyone who has been ill. A timely, perceptive and fascinating book'

Roger Kneebone, Professor of Surgical Education and Engagement Science at Imperial College London

'Encourages us to consider what it means to be human; and in doing so, how we might become better humans. A must read for every doctor, for anyone who is considering becoming a doctor, or for those who want to understand how medicine really works'

Professor Deborah Gill, Director, UCL Medical School

'A gem of wisdom as well as being so very elegantly written and entertaining. I shall be recommending it to my fellow coaches as virtually all of it apply to us as much as to clinicians' **Jenny Rogers, co-author of** *Coaching For Health: Why It Works And How To Do It*

'Using his characteristic blend of deep insight, rare candour and tongue-in-cheek humour, Launer explores a wide range of topics from the commonplace to the taboo… required reading for anyone interested in the healing arts'

Dr. Frank Jr Vertosick, author of *When the*
Air Hits Your Brain: Tales of Neurosurgery

'Funny, perceptive and varied, these essays have attracted a cult following among doctors… but there's no need to have been through a medical training to enjoy them and I'm delighted they are now available to a wider readership'

Dr Christopher Martyn, Associate
Editor, *British Medical Journal*

'An all-round excellent book, which would appeal to a wide range of healthcare professionals and students… a light-hearted way of looking at serious subjects'   **BMA Panel of Judges**

'Launer gives full voice to his own story-telling skills in this collection of short articles. He draws widely, from personal experience to imagined worlds, from evolutionary psychology to literary criticism, but he never strays far from the depth of understanding that can be gained from an interaction between patient and doctor, or learner and guide'

Professor Ronald MacVicar, Postgraduate
Dean, NHS Education for Scotland

'Launer reminds us that we as doctors need to share our vulnerabilities and be willing to explore new horizons, not just in science but about the heart and soul of what it means to be human as we journey with our patients'

Dr. Katrina Anderson, Associate Professor,
Australian National University Medical School

'Insightful, witty and above all, humane. My own practice as a doctor, and a teacher of doctors, has been enriched by reflecting on these stories'

Tim Usherwood, Professor of General Practice at
University of Sydney, and author of *Understanding*
the Consultation: Evidence, Theory and Practice

'Bursting with humor and humanity, *How Not To Be A Doctor* is a witty and engaging look at the challenges facing patients and doctors. I found myself nodding along with every page' **Dr. Matt McCarthy, author of *The Real Doctor Will See You Shortly: A Physician's First Year***

'Weaving professional and personal stories with history and theory, Launer gives us a full picture of what it means – and how it feels – to be a doctor today. Both a sober admonishment and joyful celebration of the medical profession, providing depth and colour… Fascinating'

Kevin Hazzard, author of *A Thousand Naked Strangers: A Paramedic's Wild Ride to the Edge and Back*

'A seriously funny, wickedly irreverent collection of stories. It has wise advice to those that want to be better doctors, whether young or old. Deep understanding shines through: if only every medical student could hear his advice'

Professor Glyn Elwyn, Director, Patient Engagement Research Program, Dartmouth Institute for Health Policy and Clinical Practice, USA

'Humorous, poignant, provocative, and educational… the author's opinions and anecdotes offer fresh takes on the ever changing field of medicine and how small changes in patient care have the potential to inspire radical improvements in the industry at large' *Kirkus*

'Thought-provoking and wise… Launer writes with eloquent passion, gentle humour and authority about the complexities of what is involved in becoming a good doctor… not only should it be essential reading for every medical student, but qualified doctors should be required to re-read it every year in order to reflect on the wisdom, caring and respect for patients which are contained within it' **Nudge Books**

HOW NOT
······················
TO BE A
······················
DOCTOR
······················

JOHN LAUNER

DUCKWORTH
OVERLOOK

First published in 2018 in the UK by Duckworth Overlook

LONDON
30 Calvin Street, London E1 6NW
T: 020 7490 7300
E: info@duckworth-publishers.co.uk
www.ducknet.co.uk
For bulk and special sales please contact
sales@duckworth-publishers.co.uk

British Library Cataloguing in Publication Data. A CIP record for this book
can be obtained from the British Library.

Typeset by Danny Lyle
danjlyle@gmail.com

Printed and bound in the UK by TJ International

978-0-7156-5214-5

1 3 5 7 9 10 8 6 4 2

CONTENTS

....

INTRODUCTION··XIII

1. HOW NOT TO BE A DOCTOR···1

2. STRESS TEST···5

3. PLUS ÇA CHANGE···9

4. MODERN MEDICINE···12

5. WHAT'S IN A NAME?···16

6. THE WRONG TROUSERS··19

7. CLOSE ENCOUNTERS··22

8. MENTIONED IN PASSING··26

9. ALL GREEK TO ME···30

10. ANNA O AND THE 'TALKING CURE'······································34

11. DOING THE ROUNDS···39

12. IT'S ALL IN THE BODY··43

13. DR SCROOGE'S CASEBOOK 47

14. THE ITCH 51

15. OF CHEESE AND CHOICE 55

16. LET'S TALK ABOUT SEX 59

17. MYSTERIES OF THE MALE 63

18. THE ENDURING ASYLUM 68

19. DO NOT DISTURB 72

20. BURNING YOUR RELATIVES 76

21. THE PROBLEM WITH SEX 80

22. THE ART OF QUESTIONING 85

23. HOT WATER 88

24. INTERPRETING ILLNESS 91

25. IT TAKES TWO 95

26. YELLOW NOSE SIGN 98

27. DIALOGUE AND DIAGNOSIS 102

28. BREAKING THE NEWS 106

29. CAREERS ADVICE⸺110

30. ONLY OBEYING ORDERS⸺114

31. THE ART OF NOT LISTENING⸺118

32. END OF THE ROAD⸺122

33. ESCAPING THE LOOP⸺125

34. IMPALED ON THE INVISIBLE⸺129

35. WEASEL WORDS⸺132

36. FOLK ILLNESS AND MEDICAL MODELS⸺135

37. THE FACTS OF DEATH⸺139

38. CARE PATHWAYS⸺144

39. ON KINDNESS⸺148

40. CAPABLE BUT INSANE⸺153

41. ON THE RECORD⸺157

42. CLOSE READINGS⸺161

43. MEET YOUR MICROBIOME⸺166

44. OPIUM⸺171

45. MEDICINE AS POETRY⋯⋯⋯⋯⋯⋯⋯⋯⋯⋯⋯⋯⋯⋯177

46. THE BREATHTAKINGLY SIMPLE FACTS OF LIFE⋯181

47. MONKEY BUSINESS⋯⋯⋯⋯⋯⋯⋯⋯⋯⋯⋯⋯⋯⋯⋯185

48. MEDICINE UNDER CAPITALISM⋯⋯⋯⋯⋯⋯⋯⋯190

49. MEMORIES OF THE WORKHOUSE⋯⋯⋯⋯⋯⋯⋯194

50. TAKING RISKS SERIOUSLY⋯⋯⋯⋯⋯⋯⋯⋯⋯⋯199

51. THREE KINDS OF REFLECTION⋯⋯⋯⋯⋯⋯⋯⋯203

52. BRIEF ENCOUNTER⋯⋯⋯⋯⋯⋯⋯⋯⋯⋯⋯⋯⋯⋯208

53. POWER AND POWERLESSNESS⋯⋯⋯⋯⋯⋯⋯⋯212

54. FATHERS AND SONS⋯⋯⋯⋯⋯⋯⋯⋯⋯⋯⋯⋯⋯216

FURTHER READING⋯⋯⋯⋯⋯⋯⋯⋯⋯⋯⋯⋯⋯⋯221

ACKNOWLEDGEMENTS⋯⋯⋯⋯⋯⋯⋯⋯⋯⋯⋯⋯⋯233

AUTHOR'S NOTE⋯⋯⋯⋯⋯⋯⋯⋯⋯⋯⋯⋯⋯⋯⋯⋯235

FOREWORD

....

In Search of Wisdom

John's writing has a special place on my 'wisdom shelf', in between George Bernard Shaw's The Doctor's Dilemma and Richard Asher's A Sense of Asher. In a world where medicine has become mass-produced and superficial, dictated by target-driven cookbooks, pigeon-hole labels and profit, we need a healthy dose of humanity and wisdom, and a questioning of received opinion. John Launer never disappoints.

I first met John when I was making a programme about the power of language in healing. John was passionate about the need to pay close attention to the words patients choose, the words we choose to impose on them, and the need to explore the meaning to them. "We describe it as depression. How useful is it to call it by that name? Would it be easier for you to call it lowness?" To this day, I can never impose the label of depression on anyone without asking what it means, and feels like. Words are how we change the world, and in this collection of over 50 essays, John weaves them into stories that make us stand back and reflect on what 'being a doctor' means, and whether it might sometimes be helpful not to stick to the rules or conform to the stereotype.

And there's much else besides. John covers a wide variety of topics in impressive depth, drawing on his experiences as a family doctor, family therapist, educator, English Literature graduate and patient. His passion for narrative medicine shines through, and each offering is like a personal 'conversation inviting change', the training model he has also developed. Dive in and discover the kindness of strangers, the poetry of consultations, the bias of medical discourse, the dangers of labelling, the deliberate preservation of uncertainty, the banality of evil and the perils of trying to make a human chimpanzee hybrid. I particularly enjoyed John's passionate defence of humane healthcare as it's fed through the market mincing machine. Highly recommended for doctors and patients who dare to be different, and everyone in search of the soul of medicine.

Phil Hammond
Doctor, writer, broadcaster, comic

INTRODUCTION

....

When I teach groups of other doctors, one of my favourite exercises to make people feel comfortable at the beginning of the day is to ask everyone to say what job they would have done if they hadn't chosen medicine. The answers are always surprising, and sometimes moving. For example, an anaesthetist may reveal she would have liked to be an opera singer. A surgeon discloses an 'alter ego' as a deep-sea diver. Psychiatrists speak of wanting to be foresters, pilots or dancers. Family physicians – general practitioners – name every job under the sun.

Two things are striking about these revelations. One is the passion with which they are made. In some cases there is wistfulness or regret about the road never taken. But quite often, doctors will say with pride that they have still managed to pursue these interests in one way or another, in spite of the pressures of a medical career. Being a doctor does not stop you from following any of these interests, nor indeed from playing the cello, acting in plays, painting in oils, translating novels from Japanese, keeping bees, or just about anything you can think of. Still less does it prevent you being a parent, lover, partner, carer, dreamer or indeed practically anything. Not only that, but every one of these roles and activities enriches being a doctor, whether or not your patients ever learn about them.

The essays here are all reflections, in one way or another, on the art, practice or teaching of medicine. Taken together, they set out an argument that being a doctor – a *real* doctor – should mean being able to draw on every aspect of yourself, your interests and your experiences, however remote these may seem from the medical task of the moment. I wrote them while combining several different medical and non-medical roles myself: as a general practitioner in a run-down area of London, as a therapist and tutor in a prestigious mental health institute, as an educator specialising in consultation and supervision skills, and as an author, husband and a parent of twins. The book bears the traces of all these identities, along with my own previous profession as an English teacher. It also covers topics from some of my lifelong passions, including literature, poetry, religion, psychology, art, history, travel and evolution. The essays originated in popular columns that I wrote in two medical journals over several years but are adapted here for general readers. (Where I have based an essay on other published articles or books, these are listed under "Further Reading" at the end of the book.) Some of the pieces are contemplative in tone, others are polemical, humorous, educational, fantastical, satirical or deadly serious. All serve the purpose of illustrating how nothing is really extraneous to medicine, nor medicine from anything else.

The first essay in the collection is called "How Not To Be A Doctor" and has given the book its title. It is intended to be ironic, as the essay itself explains. It illustrates how being authentic as a doctor may mean behaving in ways you were never taught, or have seen other doctors behave, but by using intuition and spontaneity. Most of all, it means drawing on what your patients bring you directly – most especially their words and stories. Patients need relief from suffering, but very often that relief comes through telling their stories, as many of the essays describe (with details altered to preserve anonymity). Doctors need to be able to hear those stories, to help people make sense of them and, wherever possible, consider how different stories might be possible. Some doctors achieve dramatic outcomes simply by being deeply knowledgeable and technically skilled. More often, I think, we succeed in our work by letting go of the habit of trying to fix everything, or fit it into categories, and instead by listening to people's stories, questioning these thoughtfully, and noticing how often things will right themselves with a little active help or even with none at all. It is a message I try to illustrate in these pages.

Another message is that we need to be able to tell our own stories as doctors too – to speak about our experiences with colleagues or, as I have done here, to set them down in writing so we can understand them better and carry on developing as practitioners. Some of the essays here literally take the form of short stories, either imaginary or autobiographical. They include accounts of when I have been a patient myself, including some episodes of illness that were life-threatening. Being a patient who is a doctor is never quite the same as being a non-medical patient, but every doctor who has gone through major illness knows how it brings more depth to the experience of practising medicine and teaching others to do so.

Throughout the book, I try to convey what practising medicine is like when you look at it as a whole person and not just as a doctor, and how different the work can be from what people imagine: more complex and contradictory, full of unexpected learning, puzzles and humour, and altogether much closer to the arts, humanities and the whole range of other human endeavours than is ever usually recognised.

1

HOW NOT TO BE
A DOCTOR

....

'How can I help you?' I asked. It isn't the way I always
open medical consultations, but I was making a video to
use when teaching junior doctors, so I thought I would be
conventional. As it turned out, it was a fortunate move. 'I'm
not sure if you really can help me,' the patient answered.
'I've seen lots of specialists, and none of them have
managed to help me so far. You see, I keep having these
funny turns...' Two weeks later, when showing the video
to a group of young doctors, I stopped the recording at this
point and asked them to write down the woman's opening
complaint. All ten of them wrote down 'funny turns'. They
were wrong, of course. The woman's opening problem was
that she wasn't sure if I could really help her. The funny
turns were at this point a lesser problem.

There were more shocks in store for the group. I spent
almost the entire consultation asking the woman about her
experience of other doctors and what they had got wrong.
I listened as dispassionately as I could, without dismissing
her catalogue of disappointment or offering any hint that I
might do any better myself. In the end I asked her what she
thought the doctors ought to have done instead. She told
me: a referral for homoeopathy or acupuncture. I asked her

which of these she would prefer. She chose the homoeopathy referral, and I said I would arrange this. As she left, I thought she was going to cry with relief.

After I had finished showing the video, one junior doctor erupted. How could I have been so incompetent – not to take a full medical history? How could I be so irresponsible, by assuming that the other doctors had all done their job properly? How could I be certain that her funny turns did not presage some terrible terminal disease? If I thought the problem was psychological, why didn't I take a decent psychiatric history instead? And how could I possibly direct her, without a clear diagnosis, towards a form of treatment that was totally unscientific, and I probably didn't believe in anyway?

A number of other doctors in the group came to my defence. Some had realised that I might have looked at the notes in advance, and that I might be willing to trust local colleagues not to have made gross errors of judgement. Others had heard the patient mention that she had gone through the mill of extensive and futile investigations several times over. One or two had noticed how the patient gave indications of an aversion to anything remotely suggesting psychological inquiry. A particularly thoughtful doctor pointed out that no intervention was without its dangers; at this stage it would probably cause the patient more risk if I started all over again, instead of just doing what she wanted. Yet their sceptical colleague remained unconvinced. How could I have behaved so... so... well, so unlike a doctor? I took the question as a compliment.

Of all professions, doctors are almost invariably the most proficient at not listening. Indeed, a friend of mine sometimes describes my educational work in consultation skills as 'remedial therapy for selective brain damage'. It is a cruel characterisation, but I do not entirely object to it. I am struck again and again by how much medical listening – even the kind that sometimes passes for being 'patient-centred' – falls desperately short of anything that one might expect from an attentive, untrained friend. Many doctors seem to tune out totally from any words or phrases that do not fit the medical construction of the world. In addition, most appear to be extraordinarily timid about going where the patient wants to lead, for fear that this will break some rule, or upset any other doctor who might hear about it.

When it comes to unexplained symptoms, I often observe doctors falling back on an impoverished list of questions such as 'Are you under any stress?' rather than displaying any true curiosity about the story itself. There are two other common consultation ploys that bring me out in an allergic reaction. One is the question 'How did you *feel* about that?' It is generally asked as the doctor leans forward in a theatrical pose of solicitousness, but with eyes glazed over in weary automatism. The question seems to go with a belief that it will elicit some nugget of truth, accompanied by a catharsis on the part of the patient. It arises, I guess, from some ghastly misreading of Freud's more minor followers, but ninety-nine times out of a hundred it is emotionally bogus. The other manoeuvre that I find equally offensive is the phrase 'It *sounds* as if…' (as in 'It sounds as if you're very upset…'). Believe me, if it's so obvious that even a doctor has noticed, it usually isn't worth saying.

Lois Shawver, a Californian therapist and teacher whom I much respect, has come up with a wonderful distinction between 'listening in order to speak' and 'speaking in order to listen'. When you listen in order to speak, you merely scan the words that patients are saying, looking for opportunities to dive in and tell them what is 'really' going on. When you speak in order to listen, you do the opposite: speaking only in order to give them more opportunities to explain their own view of the world. In a post-modern age where the authority of professional knowledge is gradually waning away, Shawver argues that we will have to learn how to speak less and listen more.

In the same vein, the radical US psychiatrist Harold Goolishian used to offer the advice: 'Don't listen to what patients mean, listen to what they say!' Quite simple really, except that, as doctors, we probably still fail to do this most of the time.

2

STRESS TEST

....

The technician came out of her room and bellowed a name at us: 'Andrew Parkinson!' There was silence as we all looked at each other sheepishly. Apart from myself, all the other people waiting in the hospital corridor were elderly women, some of them from the wards and wearing dressing-gowns. 'Andrew Parkinson!' she shouted again, this time fixing me with an accusatory look. 'John Launer?' I asked guiltily. She looked again at the form in her hand. 'Bloody hell,' she said, 'I've already done Andrew Parkinson.' She disappeared, and came back a minute later with another form. 'John Launer!' she bellowed this time, as if I might have changed my identity in the meantime.

I went into the room to have my electro-cardiogram done. She told me to strip to the waist and announced she was going to shave some small areas on my chest. No introduction, no preliminaries, no questions, no explanations, no friendly chatter to put me at my ease. 'Get up on the treadmill... I'm going to stick some pads on your chest... start to walk... now faster... *Jesus!*' She had just seen my initial reading coming out of the printer. Immediately she tore off a length of it and scurried off without another word. I could hear her anxious conversation with the junior doctor on the other side of the curtain. I wasn't very surprised when she came back to ask me if I had ever had an abnormal reading before.

It was still an odd question. My notes were in front of her, stuffed with my previous electro-cardiograms. 'Yes,' I answered. 'I've got left bundle branch block. I've had it all my life.' Incurious about my use of the technical term, she scurried away once more for another half-whispered conversation behind the curtain and then returned, apparently reassured. 'I'm a doctor,' I added – mainly to satisfy an inner need. I certainly had little expectation that it would lead to a change in her manner. She started to press buttons and the treadmill gathered speed each time. After a while I asked her if it was OK to run, as I was accustomed to jogging and found it more comfortable than having to walk very fast. She said I could, but a few minutes later she commented on how much I was perspiring, especially for someone who was used to jogging. It was a very hot day, and there wasn't a fan in the room. I refrained from pointing out that someone coming for a stress cardiogram to find out if they possibly needed heart surgery might, just conceivably, be perspiring from anxiety, even without a technician whose gift for empathy was small.

As I gathered speed, she told me that my shoulders seemed unusually tense. This was interfering with the tracing, and anyway they shouldn't be like that if I exercised regularly. I asked her how much faster the treadmill would go, and she told me there wasn't a limit. She then waited another couple of minutes before giving me the information I obviously wanted, namely whether she would stop before I got exhausted. Finally she did turn the treadmill off and I could see (by squinting sideways) that the tracing didn't appear to show any new problems. I asked if she agreed. 'Which consultant are you under?' was her response. I gave his name. 'He'll tell you at your next appointment. Here's a towel for the sweat. You can put on your clothes now, we're finished.'

The experience was excruciating, a needless act of emotional abuse where kindness would have required little effort. It was also, I suppose, no more or less cruel than thousands of such encounters that occur every day in the health service, not just with technicians, but with doctors, clerks, or just about anyone with a degree of power to exercise who lacks insight – whether for a passing moment or a whole lifetime – into what it feels like to be the other. We all have our explanations for such behaviour. They include multiple failings at the collective level: in the department, the hospital, the health service, and the nation. We also have our own preferred prescriptions for the problem, such as better pay and conditions, improved team morale, enhanced training, attractive incentives, consumer choice, becoming a more compassionate society, and so on and so forth.

The philosopher Martin Buber taught that we all live with a two-fold attitude, which he called the 'I-It' attitude and the 'I-Thou' attitude. *'If I face a human being as my Thou,'* he argued, *'he is not a thing among things, and does not consist of things.'* In the same corridor as the technician, there is a secretary who is outstandingly helpful, although presumably she shares many of the same work conditions as the technician. I know her name, her direct line and her email address. She always remembers my name, what I do, who I am seeing and why. When I contact her, she seems to operate from the premise that my request is going to be reasonable and that she will try her utmost to make sure it is met. I believe she treats everyone else in the same way. Without the active will, and the moral choice, of people like her, I suspect that all the well-meant interventions of politicians, managers and educators to improve the way patients are treated will subside into mere noise. Or to put it in Buber's words: '*All true living is meeting.*'

3

PLUS ÇA CHANGE

....

Og and Nyp sat by the fire outside the cave. Og, the older of the two medicine men, chewed hungrily at a toe taken from the mammoth that the clan had hunted down the previous day. Nyp sat quietly, staring into the dying embers of the fire.

'Call this medicine?' Og said with scorn in his voice. 'It isn't medicine as I remember it. In the old days, if a man was possessed by a evil spirit, you knew what a medicine man had to do. You consulted with the ancestors in your dreams. Then you did what they told you. You took a good flint arrowhead and a big stone, and you walloped a damn good hole into the man's skull. Next morning, he got up feeling right as rain, and the evil spirit had gone away.' Og sighed.

'And what happens nowadays?' Og spat a piece of mammoth gristle contemptuously into the ashes. 'You have to go to all the elders of the clan and ask their permission. They talk and they talk. They even ask the women what they think. Then one elder tells you that everyone these days is using bigger arrowheads and smaller stones. Another says the hole mustn't be wider than a baby's little finger. Some busybody – who wouldn't know an evil spirit if it smacked him in the face – says he's worried what the family will do if the sick person dies. Then everyone starts to prattle about the family's right to take retribution on you. Retribution! On a medicine man! Have you ever heard of anything so preposterous?'

Og reached into the pile of mammoth bones, helped himself to a collar bone, grasped it in both hands, and started to gnaw at it greedily. Nyp kept silent. He had heard Og talk like this before. He had great respect for Og and for all the medicine men of that generation. Before them, medicine had been truly Neanderthal. Now, thanks to men like Og, all of that had changed. It was impossible to imagine that mashed beetle poultices and infusions of ground sabre tooth had been totally unknown when Og had himself been a young man. How could one possibly have practised medicine without them? And when disease had decimated the clan, Nyp had seen Og in person sacrifice captives to the ancestors, with an elegance that took your breath away. But the world was changing, and men like Og could never halt progress.

'I tell you one of the worst things,' Og carried on. 'In the old days, if someone was possessed and his local medicine man couldn't expel the spirit, you used to go to the victim's cave yourself. You thought nothing of it. When did you last hear of anyone doing that? They're all too bloody self-important these days. No one does cave visits any more.'

'You could tell a lot from a cave,' he continued. 'You could see at once if the gods wanted someone to live or die. You looked at the paintings on the walls, for instance. They showed you a hell of a lot, those paintings. If all you saw was a charcoal sketch, with a few pathetic skinny rabbits, you didn't much fancy the patient's chances against an evil spirit. On the other hand, if you saw a bison hunt, painted to last a few years maybe, you knew you were in business.'

Nyp had heard the arguments before, but he wasn't convinced. He had seen these caves. They were dark and dingy. They certainly weren't the kind of places you could see enough to grind together a decent mixture of wolf dung, fresh slugs and boar sperm, or any of the other cleansing potions that people liked to swallow these days.

Og tore one last morsel off the collar bone and then hesitated between a rib and a shin bone. He chose the shin. He ate a few mouthfuls and then spoke again. 'Actually, there's something even worse than cave visits dying out. It's this new-fangled obsession with growing things. Our ancestors found plants for medicines just like they found their food. They picked things up from where the gods had left them. Nowadays you young people think you can gather the seeds and put them in the ground yourself. Then you just sit on your backsides and watch the plants come up. Tell me, do you honestly call that natural?'

'What next, I ask you?' he continued. 'Soon you'll be capturing rams and forcing them to copulate with their ewes and make lambs to order, because you can't be bothered to lift a spear to catch your dinner. What kind of life would that be?'

Nyp sighed. The old man was getting seriously carried away now, and just talking nonsense. By now, Og had finished his shin bone and was stretching his arm out again towards the pile of bones. Nyp had had enough. 'Old man,' he said, 'you eat too much mammoth meat. You ought to watch your diet more…'

4

MODERN MEDICINE

....

6.30 a.m. Woken by the alarm clock before the morning chorus. The roads are pretty clear on my way in, so for a change I manage to find a place in the main hospital car park, opposite the one reserved for the director of finance.

7.45 a.m. A working breakfast with the chief executive and medical director. Apparently they want me to re-write the section about my unit in the hospital's annual report. Bob, the chief executive, comments that it is 'too factual'. Sarah, the medical director, suggests that we should cut out a lot of the text and replace it with nice photos: she knows a good agency that provides these. I argue the toss for a while, but they manage to convince me that good PR is an absolute necessity for hospitals these days. I can't help noticing how well Bob and Sarah are getting on. I can remember when she was a medical student and used to call me 'sir', but now she is the only one apart from my mother who calls me Charlie instead of Charles. The meeting overruns, but I do hope I will get to see some patients by the middle of the morning.

8.30 a.m. I attend the first shift in this year's resuscitation training. Evidently the old mantra of 'ABC' – airways, breathing and circulation – has gone the way of the dinosaurs. The nurse running the session tells us a much longer and more helpful mnemonic, which I forget at this moment, but I have written it down in my notebook. (Apparently I am the last doctor in the hospital who still writes things down in a notebook.) Bob is at the training session too. He makes an ass of himself by saying that he would carry on doing chest compressions in preference to applying pressure to an arterial wound in someone who was haemorrhaging to death. This meeting overruns too, so I guess I shall have to fit some patients into the lunch hour.

10.00 a.m. Just in time for a meeting of the equality and diversity sub-committee, which I now chair (Sarah can be very persuasive when she puts her mind to it. When we did my job plan she had said something about me being a bit of a lightweight in the organisation: 'just seeing lots of patients and dabbling in research, but not much else'). There is a big agenda. We commission some very useful statistical reviews covering everything from consultants to our car park staff – who were accidentally left off last month's survey. This business of ethnic monitoring is another area where I used to be less than politically correct, but I got an earful about this from Bob's new young wife at a dinner party a while ago, and I am now thoroughly on message.

11.30 a.m. I get to the next meeting by the skin of my teeth. It is a mandatory fire and safety training that I signed up for several weeks ago. I feel rather ashamed of myself because I seem to have forgotten the difference between the three different types of fire extinguisher. The fire officer who does the presentation is an absolute wizard with PowerPoint, and I am a bit surprised when he mentions that he has given up active firefighting and now only does these talks. He looks quite a fit young man.

1.00 p.m. Lunch. I had expected to skip this and see some patients, but I suddenly remembered that the hospital regulator visited us earlier in the year and noticed 'a culture of comfort grazing rather than a model of healthy eating'. I decided I ought to be seen in the canteen. I hold a conversation in the queue with our education director who tells me she is introducing monthly satisfaction surveys for everyone we teach in the hospital. I have been training my juniors on the old principle of 'walking the wards' with me. I shall try to pull my socks up and go to a few meetings about educational methods. Sadly my lunch break means that I don't get time to record the morning's activities for my annual appraisal folder. I also feel rather embarrassed afterwards to discover that I missed a lunchtime meeting about disclosing poor performance in colleagues.

1.30 p.m. Most of the afternoon is taken up with the serious business of building up our patient liaison service. I am now the consultant rep on this (Sarah's influence again – what is it about that woman?) We have to interview a number of candidates from the local community to join us. It is a formidable task. Fortunately our head of human resources has already done a 'comprehensive mapping exercise of local stakeholders', and she brings along a very thorough set of guidelines about making such appointments. We take an hour just to familiarise ourselves with these, but in the end we manage to appoint some good people. Evidently there is a very robust appeals procedure for anyone who feels unfairly rejected.

4.30 p.m. All our non-medical staff are in the process of having their contracts revised: something to do with modernisation, I think, although I am not entirely clear about this. Unfortunately at the meeting itself I find that I don't really have much to contribute. My suggestion that 'Operating Theatre Assistant' remains a better term than 'Parasurgical Resource Officer Grade One' does not win favour. Apparently Bob is very keen on 'rebranding', Sarah even more so.

5.30 p.m. There is a note on my desk when I return to my office. One of my more vulnerable patients has apparently phoned up in a state and left a message with my secretary. 'He says he is pretty desperate,' she has written, 'and would be terribly grateful if you could phone as soon as possible.' I pick up the receiver, but then suddenly remember the tremendous telling-off we had all had from Sarah (and Bob) about not sticking to the Working Time Directive. Apparently our next star rating may hinge on this. Reluctantly, I replace the receiver. I shall have to make the call tomorrow – if my other commitments permit.

5

WHAT'S IN A NAME?

....

I handed a prescription to a patient last week and she asked me whether she should take it straight away *'to the apothecary'*. I thought at first that she was using the word apothecary as a joke, but she was not. At the age of ninety-seven, she was saying it without any self-consciousness – and presumably without any awareness that dictionaries have defined it as archaic for at least fifty years.

I wondered if I was witnessing the very last time that this word would ever be used in common English parlance. Doctors spend their lives listening to people, so we may be in a better position than almost anyone else to listen out for archaic words that have survived in common speech. Of course, it would be impossible scientifically to record the last usage of any word. Who could ever prove that the word 'milliner', or 'costermonger', or indeed 'apothecary' would never be spoken again?

To chronicle the very *first* usage of each word in the English language was, in its time, the biggest research project ever undertaken – the nineteenth-century equivalent of the human genome project. A doctor, as it happens, played a large part in this. When James Murray began to compile the *Oxford English Dictionary* in 1879, he solicited the help of an army of enthusiastic volunteers from around Britain. He asked

them to comb the published literature in the English tongue
since mediaeval times, and to record examples of the first
appearance of every English word, in each of its nuances. One
of Murray's most prolific correspondents, particularly for
words beginning with 'A' and 'B', was William Chester Minor,
an American surgeon resident in Berkshire.

Minor had more opportunity – and perhaps more motivation
– to go about this task than one might expect from most
surgeons. He was a traumatised survivor of the American Civil
War and suffered from paranoid schizophrenia. He was also a
convicted murderer and an inmate of Broadmoor Hospital.
Writing from a comfortable suite of rooms in the hospital
(financed from his US army pension), Minor diligently posted
his carefully researched examples to Murray in his corrugated
iron shed in Mill Hill, just north of London. Over a period of
twenty years, he sent in about twelve thousand standardised
slips. Murray was to write, 'So enormous have been Dr
Minor's contributions... that we could easily illustrate the
last four centuries from his quotations alone.' Only in Minor's
later years, when he had cut off his own penis in a fit of
post-masturbatory guilt, did his offerings cease altogether.
The entire poignant and bizarre story can be read in Simon
Winchester's book, *The Surgeon of Crowthorne*.

When my elderly patient used the word apothecary, I
naturally asked her if she meant that she ought to take her
prescription to the 'chemist'. That was ironic. I too had
betrayed my age – because of course these days chemists do
not exist either. They are known as pharmacists.

In superficial terms, apothecaries, chemists and pharmacists
are all the same. They are all people who make up medicines
and sell them. Yet at the same time, we also know that they are

quite different creatures. Each title carries a different weight, and a different set of mental associations. Apothecaries became chemists because it sounded more scientific. Chemists then wanted us to call them pharmacists because it sounded more professional. The strategy has worked, and their job status has become enhanced as a result. When you change a word, you also affect the thing it denotes.

Many philosophers nowadays argue that language not only describes reality, it also creates it. The case of apothecaries, chemists and pharmacists is a fairly straightforward example of this process at work. As doctors know, some diseases entirely vanished when we ceased to believe in their names (like neurasthenia), while new names have been conjured into existence to explain the inexplicable (such as irritable bowel syndrome). These examples of the creative power of language are fairly easy to accept, but there are some even bigger challenges to our basic medical assumptions. For example, there are compelling arguments to suggest that even words like 'asthma' cover a particular constellation of symptoms, physical signs, treatments and explanatory theories that may evaporate utterly over time. It is not just a question, say the philosophers, of having to hone down our ideas about these conditions, so that they gradually become more accurate. Our whole systems of thought about disease may in fact be no more than a set of self-referential linguistic fabrications. This isn't something we can ever hope to change as doctors; it is inherent in the nature of language itself.

This idea may seem counter-intuitive, or even absurd. That may be simply because we think in language itself, so we believe uncritically in the reality it generates. In the same way, my patient believed absolutely that she could still take her prescription to an apothecary.

6

THE WRONG
TROUSERS

....

Admittedly, I did not look like a doctor. For one thing, I had just spent ten days on the Nile in a felucca with eight fellow travellers. (Feluccas are primitive sailing boats that look romantic in travel brochures but seem less so on closer acquaintance.) Then, when we reached Luxor, I was struck by one of those acute shopping disorders that afflict tourists, and bought a pair of baggy cotton trousers with broad black and yellow stripes. I wore these for the rest of the journey, so that by the time we boarded the overnight train from Aswan to Cairo I looked like a dishevelled bumble bee.

'Is there a doctor on the train?'

The message came over the public address system, first in Arabic, then in French and finally in English. Aswan was a couple of hours behind us. I felt a strong desire to deny my profession, but in the past two weeks I had already attended almost everyone in my group for the usual unpleasant ailments that go with so-called 'adventure travel', and they all knew what I did for a living. Lurching along the corridor towards the back of the train, I found an edgy Egyptian guide attached to a party of French tourists. Judging by their dress and demeanour, they had spent considerably more on their trip than we had on ours. They raised eyebrows at my ridiculous appearance, but allowed me to enter the compartment where I met the patient, a ten-year-old boy. He was accompanied by a male guardian who could have been an uncle or perhaps a private tutor. Both guardian and boy were pale and sweaty. In the guardian's case it was no doubt from anxiety. The boy, however, had a thin racing pulse and the rigid abdomen that indicates peritonitis. I knew the likeliest cause was a burst appendix.

I explained that that the child needed urgent surgery. This provoked a frightening response. The Egyptian guide lost the few vestiges of restraint that had held her panic in check and began to shout at me. I persisted, saying that the train would need to make an unscheduled halt at Luxor to let him and his guardian go to the hospital there. At this news the guardian practically passed out, while the guide dismissed my advice completely, saying that the hospitals were bad in Luxor and the child would be much safer waiting until we reached Cairo in about eighteen hours. I said as calmly as I could that he might die within eighteen hours, and that it was beyond belief that a town the size of Luxor would not have a surgeon who could remove an appendix competently.

Various members of the French party then came in to ask for proof that I really was a doctor. Close to losing my own temper, I managed to say witheringly: 'Je suis desolé, mais je ne porte pas mes diplômes en vacances' ('I'm sorry, but I don't carry my certificates on holiday'). With bad grace, two of the French tourists finally agreed that they would discuss the matter with the guard and then dismissed me. I returned to my own carriage. I had barely finished narrating the story to my own tour party and our Dutch guide, when another announcement came over the public address system. This time it was only in

French, inquiring if there was a French doctor on the train. The stress was emphatically on the word 'français'.

I leapt up. This time, fortunately, our guide offered to come with me. He had displayed his equanimity already on the trip in various ways. I also knew that he spoke better French than me, as well as some Arabic. When we reached the boy's compartment we found, not surprisingly, that no French doctors had appeared, but a French nurse from another tour party had identified herself. She was, mercifully, an operating theatre nurse who must have seen hundreds of similar cases. Her elegance and fragrance also appeared to give her more professional authority than I had managed to convey.

Through a series of diplomatic negotiations, it was agreed that I would re-examine the boy under the appraising eyes of the French nurse. I did so. She indicated with a nod that, beneath my carnival outfit and uncouth appearance, I did seem to be a doctor, and that the signs I had elicited were grave. I supplied my name and work address to two of the more imperious Frenchmen at their request. I was unclear whether they wanted it for insurance purposes, or with the intention of suing me if I turned out to have caused them any inconvenience. Then I left.

For about six months I heard nothing, but eventually received a letter from the boy's parents in France, offering their thanks. Their son had had an emergency operation in Luxor, and had been transferred to Cairo for postoperative care, where they had joined him. His recovery had been slow and complicated, but he was now quite well. An episode that threatened to turn from farce to tragedy had ended up as one of the few occasions in my career when I can say with almost absolute certainty that I saved a life.

7

CLOSE
ENCOUNTERS

....

I sometimes get invited to run seminars on primary health care for other professions, particularly social workers and psychologists. People in these professions can have odd ideas of what primary health care is and does, and even odder stereotypes about GPs. One of the ways I tackle these stereotypes is to ask seminar members to get into pairs and tell each other about encounters with GPs. I ask them to exchange one story about a recent professional encounter, followed by one story about a personal encounter when they have visited a GP's surgeries as a patient, carer or parent.

A striking contrast often emerges between the two sets of stories. Tales of professional encounters usually centre on the frustrations of trying to contact GPs during busy clinics, or the mutual incomprehension that can occur when trying to discuss a shared case or elicit some information from a GP. The personal stories, on the other hand, generally have quite a different tone. They speak of longstanding, trusting and even tender relationships with family doctors. They testify to people's capacity to tolerate all the huge and conspicuous inadequacies of general practice in exchange for the things they value: a listening ear, a warm touch, some blunt advice, and the ability to display friendliness without an inappropriate claim to friendship. Inviting people to reflect on the contrast between their personal and professional encounters can then lead people to hold a subtler and less critical view of primary care.

Another exercise I use is even more fruitful. It is to ask people to share memories of the GPs they saw when they were children. Almost invariably, people recall their childhood family doctors with respect and fondness. However, this can be a very powerful exercise, so it is unfair to set this exercise without being prepared to reflect on one's own recollections. And so I find myself casting my mind back to the three GPs of my own childhood and adolescence: Dr Newman, Dr Tanner, and Dr Dean.

Dr Newman was a refugee from Nazi Germany. We used to go into his consulting room from the waiting room when a red light came on, but afterwards we went out straight through the back door into his yard, so you never knew how much time he spent alone between patients. Sometimes he asked you how many people there still were in the waiting room. If you told him the number was large, he would groan. My mother came from Vienna – in the same era and for the same reason – so they spoke together in German. Dr Newman dispensed lots of practical advice, and once told my mother to go out and buy a fridge, which she did. He was famous in our family for always claiming to suffer from whatever ailment you came with. *'Das hab ich auch!'* he would say: *'I've got that too!'* The favourite family story about him told of the day my mother went to him with a foot complaint. He took off his shoes and socks, and then put his feet up on the desk to prove his claim. After that, we changed our doctor. As an adult, I can guess at the reasons why his relentless claims for sympathy for his own suffering became intolerable for my mother.

We moved to Dr Tanner. For some reason I am entirely unable to explain, I am quite certain she was a Roman Catholic. She was very well spoken, and there was an aura about her that she was 'a cut above' the area of London where we lived and she practised. (How can a child of two continental Jewish refugees have been so aware of English accents, religious denominations and class? Yet it seems I was.) She was frail-looking, tense and pale, and I connect that in my mind with her departure after only three or four years, although that connection may only be a fantasy. She was kind, and I felt safe with her.

She was replaced by Dr Dean, whose most striking feature to a nine-year-old boy was the prodigious quantity of hair growing from his ears. He was Indian, and my adult self deduces that he was a Sikh, although he did not wear a turban. One of the most magical things he used to do was to reach into the drawers of his desk for samples that visiting pharmaceutical reps had just left for him. He would then hand them over to my mother to try out on my eczema. As a result, I tried out hydrocortisone cream for the first time. Hence I was able to throw away the thick tar ointments that had befouled my bedclothes for years, and the bandages I had had to wear under my trousers at school. I loved the presence, smell and feel of Dr Dean: burly, squidgy and comforting all at the same time. The last time I saw him was in late adolescence for a medical before I went off to teach in Kenya for my gap year. I was convinced he was going to discover the extensive cancer I had been concealing for years. He didn't, and so my trip went ahead. On my return from Africa, I went to a university doctor who told me my fears were ungrounded. I had been suffering all through my teens from swollen glands in my armpits and groin as the consequence of my eczema.

I have no idea if these three numinous figures influenced my eventual decision (halfway through university) to become a doctor and later to be a GP. But I recognise in these memories – and the memories evoked in my seminars – a truth that as doctors we often ignore or forget. The experience that most patients have of doctors is a sensual, affective and aesthetic one. Moral and cognitive judgements may sometimes displace their consciousness of this, but they cannot obliterate it. In all our professional encounters, the acuity that our patients had as children still persists.

8

MENTIONED IN
PASSING

....

For twenty years, my main place of work was in Edmonton. As London suburbs go, Edmonton is definitely not chic. Some Londoners have never even heard of it. Others only know it as the place where most of London's garbage is incinerated. Most simply have a vague impression of it as somewhere that flashes by on the North Circular Road. Essentially, Edmonton is on the way from somewhere to somewhere else.

Edmonton is transitional in other ways too. Few of our patients were actually born here. Even fewer dreamed of living out the rest of their days in Edmonton. Some moved there in order to buy their first property, and their greatest hope was to move out of London altogether, to the leafy vales of Hertfordshire. Others arrived as refugees, but once they know London better, they had no wish to stay in Edmonton any more than they wanted to return to Kosovo, Somalia or Kurdistan. For them too, Edmonton was a staging post.

Perhaps it is no coincidence that Edmonton was once a staging post in a quite literal sense. Before the railway came, turning Edmonton from a pretty Middlesex village into a characterless London suburb, the stage coaches stopped here on their way out of the city and into Hertfordshire. Ironically, many Londoners over the centuries must have taken their first breath of country air around Edmonton Green.

Back in its village days, Edmonton had many literary connections, especially around the turn of the nineteenth century. Curiously, nearly all of these are of medical or psychiatric interest. One of Britain's most popular poets, John Keats, was apprenticed to a Dr Hammond in Church Street. Keats never completed his training, and later he moved to Hampstead. Nevertheless, on the site of Hammond's surgery in Edmonton there is now a Keats Parade with a Keats Pharmacy. Nearby, there is a Keats Surgery. The North Middlesex Hospital, which squats like a carbuncle on the North Circular Road, boasts a Keats Ward. Keats could hardly complain we have forgotten him.

Keats is not Church Street's only literary figure from that time. In the churchyard itself is the grave of Charles Lamb and his sister Mary – known to generations of children as the authors of *Tales from Shakespeare*. Their original reason for leaving London was that Mary had murdered their mother while in the grip of delusions. Astonishingly for the time, she was not incarcerated but allowed to stay in the care of her brother. They first moved to Enfield, but then came to Edmonton to obtain medical treatment for Mary's worsening schizophrenia. Alas, the task of being her carer told on Charles. He took to the bottle and eventually died from the consequences of a fall. Mary never again recovered her sanity.

As well as figuring in these literary lives, Edmonton appears in one of England's best known comic poems: the ballad of John Gilpin. The ballad tells of a luckless London merchant who wanted to join his family at the Bell Inn in Edmonton in order to celebrate his wedding anniversary. The celebration never happens. Through a farcical series of frights and mishaps, Gilpin is unable to stop his horse galloping past Edmonton into Hertfordshire, and then galloping straight back into London. The ballad is obviously poking fun at its hero, but could it be making a point about Edmonton as well? One is left wondering what is it about the place that has this effect on humans and animals alike.

The ballad's author, William Cowper, was never a resident of Edmonton, but he must have known it well as a passing place. He has since been adopted as an honorary Edmontonian: the Bell was renamed the John Gilpin Bell, and there is now a John Gilpin Ward at the North Middlesex Hospital too.

Cowper himself led a life in many ways similar to Mary Lamb's. He spent most of it in the grip of a terrifyingly severe depression. Like Mary Lamb, he had a devoted carer for many years – in his case a widowed woman friend called Mrs Unwin. He too sank into permanent despair once his carer died. Before that, he wrote some of the most poignant descriptions we have of melancholy and paranoia. In his letters, Cowper explained that he wrote John Gilpin and many of his other poems in order to keep insanity at bay. He translated the whole of Homer not once but twice, doing a certain number of verses each day to fend off 'Mr Bluedevil'.

Unlike Keats, Cowper is no longer popular. You can go into just about any second-hand book shop in England and pick up a long-discarded volume of his verse for fifty pence. Sadly it is unlikely to include his Homer, which is a masterpiece and possibly the greatest of all the English translations. I would take Cowper's complete works to my desert island in preference to Keats's poetry any day. But then I have always rebelled against fashion – which is probably why I have a soft spot for Edmonton after all these years.

9

ALL GREEK TO ME

....

The consultation was difficult from the start. The patient appeared to speak some English, but it was barely adequate. She had come into my surgery clutching two pieces of paper. She opened the first, which was a calendar of the past year. There were circles around almost every date, some in red ink and others in black. Some of the dates were annotated in her handwriting, in her native Greek. She was evidently trying to tell me about her periods. They were too long or too short, too frequent or not frequent enough – I was not sure which. I wondered if she was trying to get pregnant, or perhaps trying not to get pregnant. So far, it was hard to know.

She opened the second piece of paper. It was a picture from an ultrasound scan. I thought I could make out the womb, and an ovarian cyst on the right side (no great technical feat here, as they were labelled in English for some reason). The cyst looked as if it was probably a fairly small and innocent one, but I was very far from certain.

She was flustered. She wanted to explain lots of things to me, and I guessed that she probably wanted me to explain lots of things to her too. She hadn't let us know in advance that she might need a lot of time or someone to translate. Reluctantly, I phoned through to the office and asked them to get a Greek interpreter on the line. By the time the call came through I was already running late, and I knew that my decision would make the whole session, and my mood, foul.

Having a phone interpreter made things a bit better, but not hugely. At least we managed to establish that the woman's periods were infrequent but prolonged. Also she had no wish to get pregnant, and she gasped with horror when the interpreter explained that I hadn't been sure. Apart from that, the story got more confused. Through the interpreter, she explained that she was sure it was the cyst that was making her periods too long. A professor of gynaecology in Athens had told her so. Every time she had a long period, she explained, he used to give her injections of antibiotics to bring it to an end.

There ought to be a word for the stories that patients tell about their previous encounters with doctors, especially the very common kind like this that have no perceptible relationship to recognisable diseases or familiar treatments, and that pile up 'non sequiturs' nightmarishly on each other. I wasn't sure whether (a) the patient had misunderstood what happened in Greece, (b) there was something I didn't know about single cysts, prolonged periods and antibiotics, or (c) the Greek doctor there was a quack. I got even hotter under the collar at the thought of trying to unscramble the rapidly escalating muddle.

There are consultations that go very well and harmoniously and leave you with a nice warm feeling about what a caring and attentive doctor you are. There are other consultations where you wonder why you chose medicine as a career. Suddenly, you recall all those trivial and arbitrary circumstances that led to such apparent inevitability, and you find your mind wandering to all the paths in your life that you never took: novelist,

31

traveller, philanderer, tycoon. Fighting off such thoughts with diminishing success, I tried desperately to ask a few more questions through the interpreter to establish even the most tenuous commonality between this woman's understanding and mine. Each question failed. Each answer seemed to open up a new and previously unimagined conceptual chasm.

Reader, I lost it. I stopped remotely trying to understand her problem, let alone to solve it. Instead, I hectored her (it certainly felt to me like hectoring) about the impossibility of dealing with complex problems in haste. I reproached her (it certainly felt like a reproach) with giving me inadequate notice of the time and facilities that would be needed. I confronted her (it certainly felt like a confrontation) with the fact that much of her story seemed either incomprehensible or implausible to me. I rounded off this tirade (it certainly felt like a tirade) by pointing out that I wasn't her regular doctor anyway and it would make far more sense to book next time with the doctor who knew her best, giving enough notice to the receptionists, and so on and so forth...

I knew already that this was the kind of consultation that would later leave me wincing with secret shame at the recollection of my lack of professionalism towards this patient, let alone the appalling impression I must have created on the interpreter. This was certainly not an encounter that I could ever report to colleagues. And so it would no doubt have remained, had it not been for her response: 'You have been very kind, doctor, and I should like to see you next time.'

I was speechless. I would certainly not have named kindness among the emotions I had been struggling with during the previous twenty minutes. How on earth could she have perceived me as kind? Perhaps she been struck by my willingness, albeit grudgingly, to call in the aid of an interpreter. Maybe she experienced my prolonged ranting at her about resources as entirely proportionate to the scale of her need. Or was she responding to something rather more intangible?

Time and again, doctors have to re-learn that what patients seem to value in us is not usually technical expertise and certainly not charm. It may be the thing that we try our hardest to avoid: being ourselves.

10

ANNA O AND THE
'TALKING CURE'

....

'At the time of her falling ill (in 1880) Fräulein Anna O was twenty-one years old.' Thus begins one of the most famous of all medical case histories. Its author was Dr Josef Breuer. A kind, cultivated and generous man, Breuer was one of the most distinguished physicians of his time. He was also an eminent physiologist and discovered which nerves affect respiration, as well as the how the balance apparatus in the ear works. For some years he engaged a young man named Sigmund Freud to work in his laboratory at the University of Vienna, and it was Freud who eventually managed to persuade him to publish the details of Anna's illness and treatment.

Anna, according to Breuer, 'had hitherto been consistently healthy and had shown no signs of neurosis during her period of growth. She was markedly intelligent, with an astonishingly quick grasp of things and penetrating intuition. She had great poetic gifts, which were under the control of a sharp and critical common sense.' In spite of these attributes, Breuer reported, Anna fell prey, during her father's final illness and in the months after his death, to the most appalling symptoms of paralysis in three out of her four limbs, together with a succession of other distressing psychiatric symptoms. At different times these included weakness, inability to turn her head, double vision, a nervous cough, loss of appetite, hallucinations, agitation, mood swings, abusive and destructive behaviour, amnesia, excessive sleepiness, tunnel vision and abnormalities of speech ('She no longer conjugated verbs,' Breuer recorded, 'and eventually she used only infinitives, for the most part incorrectly formed from weak past participles'). Among her symptoms, she was at one time unable to speak in her native German, but could still read both French and Italian, translating them aloud into English as she did so. During part of her illness, she was unable to recognise or accept food from anyone except her physician, who spent somewhere in the region of a thousand hours with her between April 1881 and June 1882. She was able to satisfy herself of his identity only by holding his hands.

As described by Dr Breuer, his treatment of Anna gradually developed through three stages, as he responded to Anna's own apparent wishes. In the first stage, he recognised that she could relieve her distress by making up and telling fairy tales, 'always sad and some of them very charming' – and he encouraged her to do so. She herself called this activity 'chimney sweeping' or her 'talking cure' (this would later become a famous description of psychoanalysis). In the second stage, Breuer was able to hypnotise Anna every morning, sometimes by holding up an orange, in order to help her to remember some of the painful emotions she had gone through when her father was dying. Each evening Breuer would return and Anna would recount, with vivid emotion, the exact events from precisely one year previously. In the final stage, Anna began to add to these accounts a description of the various occurrences that had evidently triggered each of her hysterical symptoms during the previous year. As she did so, the relevant symptom itself would disappear. For example, on recalling her disgust at seeing a dog drink from a lady companion's glass of water a year before, she was suddenly able to drink once more, having for some time been able to quench her thirst only by eating fruit such as melons.

Breuer's history of Anna O has given rise to a tremendous amount of debate. There seems to be much uncertainty about the true extent of Anna's improvement following the treatment. We know that she was admitted to a sanatorium shortly after her apparent 'cure', still in a very disturbed state – although in later life she became a distinguished social worker and a noted campaigner for women's rights (under her real name of Bertha Pappenheim). Freud himself was the first to criticise Breuer for his naïveté, in particular for ignoring Anna's fairly obvious sexual feelings towards her physician. Breuer himself, if not actually infatuated with Anna, certainly seems to have been drawn into a kind of 'folie à deux', accepting her behaviour and her self-prescribed cures at face value, and discounting the effect of his own intense interest on her performance. It has also been suggested that Anna's theatrics drew heavily on the contemporary craze in Vienna for stage hypnotism. For many modern readers, it may be quite hard to avoid the impression of an annoying young woman running rings around a rather suggestible doctor.

However, it may be worth applying some historical sensitivity to the case history. If Anna's hysteria appears to us now as a form of outrageous fabrication, it may be for the simple reason that she had lost the capacity either to know the truth or to tell it. In addition, within her own cultural world such 'mad' behaviour was one of the few permissible forms of protest open to young women who felt stultified by their family and social circumstances. (There was opposition, for example, to girls receiving secondary education, on the grounds that it might lead to demands for women to enter the university.) Seen from this kind of perspective, her girlish determination to engage her physician with a bizarre drama of symptoms and remedies does indeed represent a shocking state of mind, and a desperate plea for help.

For his part, when Breuer approached Anna's bedside with an apparently obsessive interest in the tiniest details of her behaviour, he was displaying the most enlightened stance available to a medical man of his time, not to mention a great deal of patience and devotion. What Breuer did was in fact utterly original in relation to any form of mental distress: he listened not only in order to establish a diagnosis, but also to effect a treatment. Freud, for all his reservations about the case, realised how radical this was, and drew on it for the basis of his own talking cure. If, with hindsight, we regard Breuer's view of these events (not to mention Freud's) as somewhat selective and self-promoting, this may be no more the case than with many other scientific advances at that time – and since.

We now live in a world that is united by the idea that talking does indeed cure. Whether as doctors or therapists, our daily experience is that letting people talk does make a difference. Few if any psychotherapists these days believe, like Breuer, that prompting patients to recall trivial events from the recent past will alleviate psychological symptoms. Most believe that talking works because it provides people with a means of creating a coherent narrative from disconnected symptoms, events, memories and thoughts in the context of a relationship with someone compassionate and attentive. Whether this relationship lasts for a single medical consultation or a long course of therapy, it may help to correct some of the hurt done by less well-attuned relationships, or by significant losses and setbacks, and to make sense of them. What is particularly interesting is that a growing amount of research by neuroscientists and psychiatrists working together now suggests that such processes may bring about demonstrable changes in the brain. If this is true, we may have come full circle. It would no doubt have delighted Dr Josef Breuer, physician and physiologist, who held Bertha Pappenheim's hands, listened to her fairy stories and took them seriously.

11

DOING THE ROUNDS

....

One of the greatest figures in the history of British hospitals in the twentieth century was not a doctor, but a former steelworker from Glasgow who later became a social worker and then a film maker. His name was James Robertson.

Robertson started his researches into paediatric wards in Britain in 1948. At that time, sick children were routinely separated from their parents for long periods of time. Having parents in hospital was regarded as disruptive, and staff were upset hearing children cry when mothers arrived or left. Visits were restricted and in some cases forbidden. Here, for example, is a list of the visiting times in some of London's main hospitals from around that time, published in a survey in the Spectator:

> Guys Hospital, Sundays 2–4 p.m.; St Bartholomew's, Wednesdays 2–3.30 p.m.; St Thomas's, first month no visits, but parents could see their children asleep 7–8 p.m.; Westminster, Wednesdays, 2–3 p.m.; West London, no visiting; Charing Cross, Sundays, 2–3 p.m.; London Hospital, under three years old, no visits but parents could see through partitions, over three years old, twice weekly.

The story of Robertson's campaign to change this state of affairs sheds no glory on hospitals, doctors or the British establishment. His meticulous researches into the effects of separation on children – distrust, rejection, bed-wetting, soiling, anxiety and rages – were dismissed as sensational. The film he made with his wife Joyce to demonstrate these effects was shown at the Royal Society of Medicine in 1952 to unanimous derision, and to accusations of rigging. BBC producers blocked his attempts to present it on television. When they finally relented in 1961 and allowed him to show some excerpts, Robertson defied their orders by turning to the live camera to explain that parents had a legal right to stay with their children regardless of any 'official' rules. His courage inspired a group of mothers to form the National Association for the Welfare of Children in Hospital, one of the most effective pressure groups ever. As a result of their work, there are probably no paediatric wards in Britain nowadays with restrictions on parental visiting.

I find Robertson's story inspiring but I am also outraged by it. The list of hospital visiting times, in particular, is heartbreaking. It makes me go hot and cold with anger, misery and a retrospective sense of helplessness. The emotional effects of such institutionalised brutality are too painful to hold in the imagination. How on earth can it have happened? How can people have ever believed that it was a good thing? How could doctors and nurses have been so blind to the distress they were causing, and so uncritical of themselves?

The answer, of course, is that the rules were familiar, and familiarity breeds conformism. As Robertson found, protests against convention can invite ridicule, particularly from the medical profession. We also need to remind ourselves of innumerable other examples of social practices that were considered humane for considerable periods of time, but that now fill us with horror – including slavery, workhouses, and large mental asylums in remote rural locations.

Which brings us, somewhat uncomfortably, to the question of whether there are any current practices that doctors now accept with complacency, but ought to regard as similarly grotesque. My own nomination for such a practice would be the ward round.

Before you accuse me of descending from the sublime to the ridiculous, let me explain that I have been a hospital in-patient myself several times, so I know from experience what it feels like to lie horizontally, in ill-fitting hospital pyjamas, while small groups of fully dressed and vertical doctors (some of whom have never introduced themselves) stand over you briefly to conduct a consultation about matters of life and death, within earshot of patients in neighbouring beds. More distressingly, I have seen my wife subjected to the same humiliation by groups of mainly male colleagues, while I was dismissed from her bedside. And when my parents were alive, I observed each of them reduced to a state of humiliation, bewilderment, and more or less utter disempowerment each time they were in hospital and were victims of this uncaring but unchallengeable ritual.

In all these situations, I have wondered how it could still be permissible for patients to pass through their entire admission to hospital without ever having the basic human dignity of one-to-one meetings with their doctors, sitting in a private space such as a ward office or day room, properly clothed if possible, and with family members present if they wished. I also find it dispiriting that some consultants manage to complete their entire careers without ever engaging in a single medical encounter of this kind with an in-patient (except possibly in their private practices). I am puzzled as to why hospital teams cannot allocate one main doctor to each in-patient so that this can happen.

From the perspective of general practice, confidential encounters between a single doctor and a patient or family are the cornerstone of good medical and emotional care. There seems no reason, beyond professional convention and convenience, why this cannot happen in hospitals too. Even frail and elderly patients can in most cases be helped to dress properly and to come alone into an office – with the help of a wheelchair if necessary – so that they can disclose their fears and articulate their questions in relative dignity. For the few who cannot, it is perfectly possible for any doctor to draw up a chair to the bedside on each visit. The medical team can of course still meet, as some already do, to discuss the 'case' quite separately from arranging for one sole doctor to meet the actual person face to face.

I wonder if we will have to wait for a latter-day James Robertson so that this happens, or whether our own profession could seize the initiative in bringing the time-honoured but demeaning practice of ward rounds to an end.

12

IT'S ALL IN
THE BODY

....

'You want me to see a physician?' The patient was clearly aghast. 'A physician?'

Dr Barton sighed inwardly. He wondered, yet again, why the patients he saw in his psychiatric clinic so often found this suggestion unacceptable. The stigma attached to physical illness was still very great, in spite of all that the medical profession and the media had done to educate the public. Almost daily, he saw patients like this. They were only too happy to confess their deep-seated feelings of insecurity, or their unmanageable sexual desires. But they would nearly all conceal from him if, for example, they had had their gall bladders removed, or had ever taken painkillers. The sense of shame was too great.

'The fact is,' Dr Barton explained patiently, 'we've investigated your symptoms very thoroughly. You've scored zero on the depression inventory. According to the interpersonal functioning scale, you're coping superbly. It's the same with all your other results. We really need to look at some other kind of explanation...'

'But I don't understand. Surely you're not suggesting it's all in the body?'

It was a familiar response. As a psychiatrist, Dr Barton heard it almost every day. For each patient who was grateful to receive news of normal results like this, there were ten whose faces dropped when they learned that they were mentally healthy. It seemed as if they placed all their hopes on being told they had something like manic depression or anorexia. They regarded the lack of a firm psychiatric diagnosis as a rejection. The implication that they might have a physical problem instead was seen as a positive insult.

It must be tough being a physician, he reflected. As a high flyer, he had never really considered internal medicine as a serious option in his own career. Indeed, his professor of psychiatry at medical school had warned him not to squander his talents on a backwater specialty like cardiology. A few of his friends had gone on to deal with bodily problems; they were strange folk on the whole, but you probably had to be strange if you wanted to spend your life mucking around with problems like blood pressure and breathlessness. He recognised that physicians did perfectly respectable work in their own way. He was just pleased he was doing something so much more prestigious and lucrative.

'Please don't misunderstand me,' he continued to explain. 'I'm not questioning your symptoms. I certainly don't think you're making them up. It's just that we could waste a lot of your time doing more and more tests and still coming up with the same answer: you're basically sane.'

'So what exactly are you suggesting, then?'

Dr Barton took a deep breath. 'Look, I'd really like you to see a colleague of mine called Dr Kreinschpindl…'

'And with a name like that, I suppose he's a physician?'

'Well in a sense he is, but he's a special kind of physician, who tries to help people like you when we can't find anything wrong mentally. He works with a team of colleagues from all sorts of fields: lab scientists, physiotherapists and so on. They nearly always come up with something. We call it our Pain Clinic.'

'But I keep telling you, I'm not in any pain.'

'Not consciously, no – but that's the whole problem. The body can work in strange ways. Sometimes people think they're miserable, when the real problem is that they've got pain all over. I've sent lots of people to our Pain Clinic and they've often been every bit as sceptical as you. They didn't think for one moment that their problem might be a rheumatic one, for example, or neurological. But once they see Dr Kreinschpindl they come away realising they were actually in tremendous physical discomfort. They've been very grateful.'

In private, Dr Barton actually had some reservations about Frank Kreinschpindl. He was a real oddball, even for a physician. His conviction that everything could be reduced to physical illness bordered on the fanatical. Yet, unusually for a physician, he had made a considerable name for himself in the academic world. He had published a ground-breaking study of a group of patients who were convinced they had personality disorders, until Kreinschpindl showed that they all had nutritional deficiencies, multiple allergies or widespread fungal infections. Kreinschpindl's results were impressive too. Dr Barton would never forget a young woman he had seen who thought she was agoraphobic, until Kreinschpindl confined her to a wheelchair and put her on massive doses of steroids. She had never looked back since.

'Well, it doesn't sound as if you're giving me much choice. So how soon can I see this... this physician?'

The patient spat out the last word with the usual mixture of fear and contempt. However, Dr Barton recognised it was a victory of sorts. At least he could now discharge the patient from his clinic, even if it turned out that Kreinschpindl could do little to help.

As he drew the consultation to a close, he began to wonder what the next patient would be like. He glanced at the clinic list and gave another sigh, but this time it was one of relief. He really was in luck. The next patient was a woman he knew well and always looked forward to seeing, someone he regarded as having real insight and integrity. And she suffered from the kind of problem that would inspire sympathy and commitment in any doctor: paranoid delusions.

13

DR SCROOGE'S
CASEBOOK

....

'*Dear Doctor*,' I wrote to the admitting doctor at the local hospital when the visit was finally over, '*This woman appears to have a perforated lung …*'

I had visited the patient in question three days before Christmas. I had just completed my last work session before going off for two weeks' break with my family. There was one home visit to do, then Christmas lunch with the team, and my work would be finished for the year. I set off in the car to do the visit, but the traffic was backed up for nearly a mile, and I decided to turn round so as not to miss the lunch. No matter, I thought, I could do the visit on the way home when the traffic might be lighter. It sounded as though the patient only needed a quick eyeballing anyway.

I had already talked on the phone that morning to the care manager who had asked for the visit. The patient was a woman in her sixties who lived alone, drank alcohol heavily, and frequently had falls. The manager was concerned about an escalation in the drinking and the falls, with the woman apparently looking even more battered and bruised than normal as a result. However, the manager's main concern was that the patient's accommodation was clearly unsuitable. The neighbours were protesting about the loud drinking bouts, and they were afraid that she would injure herself. In the new year, the manager said, we would have to get her moved to somewhere safer and more suitable. I noted the phrase 'in the new year' with relief. The patient was not one of mine anyway, so the long-term arrangements would be someone else's problem. I could nip in and out of the house, check that the woman was mobile and no more incoherent than usual, and still get home by mid-afternoon.

The traffic was no better at the second attempt. I cut up a couple of cars in order to change lanes and gain a few seconds' advantage. When I rang the bell at the flat, the woman pulled aside the curtain in her bedroom and signalled to me that she would come to the door and I should wait. She then managed to totter round to let me in, although she asked for my arm to lean on as we walked back to the bedroom. The place was bleak and disgusting, and I had to fight a feeling of being repelled by the woman herself. To save time, I asked her a few curt questions and checked her over while I did so. She had a swollen face that I assumed was the consequence of having two massive black eyes, but she managed to open both eyes when I asked her to. Her limbs were covered in bruises, and the skin had been sheared off her knees, with old slough in places. However, she told me she had made a cup of tea earlier and had drunk it. She also kept saying something about chicken and bacon, but I could not follow it. Her speech was honking and slurred, seemingly not just from the alcohol but perhaps from some other, lifelong impairment.

By now I was feeling impatient. I was angry about the traffic, angry about my vanishing afternoon, and angry with the colleague I was covering for (even though he had swapped the session at my request so I could get away). I had my own

48

priorities, and making sense of the chicken and the bacon was not one of them – I wanted my holiday to start. Her condition was shocking, but no doubt had been so for a long while. She was sufficiently mobile to get to her phone or her front door. The care manager would visit again tomorrow in any case. I was reaching the point where I had decided to quit the flat and resume my life unimpeded by the needs of others, including people like this woman who live at the margins.

As an afterthought, I decided to check her chest. In the midst of talking about chicken and bacon she had mumbled something about being short of breath, but I had paid no attention because I was only really concerned about her mobility. Now it occurred to me that she might have broken some ribs in a fall as well, so I reluctantly asked her to take off her blouse. As I pressed on her sides, I felt something I have only ever felt once before: a sensation similar to treading freshly fallen snow underfoot. They taught us at medical school that it could be a sign of a perforated lung – something you could get from a broken rib.

At first she refused to go into hospital. The chicken and bacon, it turned out, were going to be part of a Christmas lunch that she was looking forward to and was due to arrive from 'Meals on Wheels'. For various reasons, it took another hour to set up all the arrangements to get her admitted, including half a dozen phone calls and involving a further journey to the surgery and back to meet up with the care manager. The traffic was no better this time either.

As I finally composed the letter for the ambulance crew to take up to hospital with the patient, I reflected on how I had managed to reduce this turbulent experience into the clipped, logical and efficient language of medicine. Would the hospital doctor who read my referral letter, I wondered, guess at the larger picture: the squalor in which some of our patients live, the pressures that lead us to cut corners, and the guardian angel who looked after me when alienation and meanness of spirit threatened to take me over.

14

THE ITCH

....

I have just run the hot water tap and put my hands underneath it, with the water as hot as I could bear, for as long as I could bear. The water was probably hotter than most people could stand, certainly beyond the temperature to cause pain. That was why I did it. I have been trying to reach the pain threshold in order to 'crack' the itch from my eczema.

To its sufferers, eczema is not principally a disease of appearance. It is a disease of itch. The itch is at times intolerable. Only hot water close to boiling point will crack it. Almost everyone with eczema knows this. It is part of the subjective knowledge that binds us as sufferers: a knowledge that lies in a quite different dimension from anything you will ever read in textbooks.

I have had eczema all my life. It is hard to be certain how much of my disposition as an adult is due to eczema and how much to other parts of my inheritance from biology and biography. But it would be odd if it did not have its inner representations in habits of thought, feeling, images and relationships. From what I know of myself, I would say that eczema and the struggle to live with it earlier on in my life have shaped me to a significant degree. Perhaps this is true of everyone who has had significant illness in childhood.

Nowadays my eczema is limited to my hands and is entirely manageable, but as a child I had eczema in many places, including the inside of my elbows, behind my knees and around my ankles. Many of my memories of childhood are memories of disordered skin sensation: the itch itself, the incessant and futile struggles to resist it, the almost erotic release of surrendering to it, and the unbearable tension of trying to scratch enough to relieve the itch without gouging down to the flesh. Often, it was impossible to sustain the tension. I would give way to a frenzy of scratching, often privately in the toilet where no one could see what I was doing. The frenzy would lead in turn to other sensations: the immediate rawness of the newly weeping patches, followed in due course by the downright pain of hardened, stiffened and cracking skin. The rawness was usually accompanied by shame, the stiffness by a kind of despair.

I was born in the days before the steroid ointments like hydrocortisone that are commonly used nowadays, so the memory of the condition itself is mixed with the pungent and sometimes brutal treatments that were in fashion at the time. At night I had cotton gloves tied on to my hands in vain attempts to limit the damage from scratching, and at times my arms were put in cardboard tubes overnight to prevent me getting to my elbows. Later, I was taken to the old skin hospital in the west end of London for radium treatment, until this was found to be a good way of inducing leukaemia.

Like almost every other disease, eczema is an interactional condition as well as an intrinsic one. When my parents fought, which they did a great deal, I would itch and scratch more. My scratching and itching probably exacerbated their bad moods and sense of helplessness as well. Because of its shocking visibility, eczema is a social condition too. At primary school, the only girl I could dance with was a red-haired girl I did not much care for, who was herself afflicted with dry and scaly skin. She had no other choice of partner either. Ironically, I found her skin particularly repulsive because its appearance and texture was not the same as mine.

At least the teachers in that school let me cover some of my worst patches with long trousers. When I started at secondary school, I shivered in grey flannel shorts while other boys stared at my legs and wondered (or so I thought) what terrible diseases they might catch from me. In the swimming pool and on the rugby field, I contrived to keep the backs of my legs out of people's sight lines as much as I could. Scratching, as always, still went on out of view. Probably very few people noticed the powdering of dry skin flakes on cubicle floors, and almost certainly they would not have known what to make of it.

A few years later, I discovered how to use my understanding of eczema productively. While I was a medical student, I joined together with about fifty other sufferers and parents to establish the National Eczema Society. In time, I sat on its research and scientific committees, and I am now proud to be one of its first honorary life members. At a more mundane level, I also take pride in being able to explain the minutiae of skin care to eczematous patients or their parents. For example, I know how important it is to be meticulous about exactly how to apply moisturisers – on newly washed skin that is still slightly damp. I also know how pointless and infuriating it is to be told 'Don't scratch!' I sometimes advise parents to tell their children 'Don't itch!' If nothing else, the paradoxical injunction may stop people in their tracks and invite them to respect the compulsiveness of the condition.

The corollary of this knowledge is an awareness of how vast my ignorance must be of the subjective experience that lies behind all the diseases that I see at work but have never suffered from myself. At least that ignorance is a handicap I share with every other doctor.

15

OF CHEESE
AND CHOICE

....

I am standing by the cheese cabinet in our local supermarket. (This is poetic licence, you understand. I am actually sitting at my computer, but my recent supermarket experience is so vivid that I am reliving it.) I am in a state of high anxiety. In front of me are uncountable types of cheese. There is Canadian, Irish, Welsh, New Zealand and English. There is mild, mature, extra-mature, vintage and farmhouse. There is low fat, full fat – presumably 'high fat' would be a marketing disaster – and vegetarian. There are special cheeses in expensive waxy paper, or in the kind of customised black rind you see in Dutch markets. There is also 'value' cheese with a logo that allows you to proclaim your penury or your meanness. These are the varieties of Cheddar alone.

Faced with such an obscene superfluity of Cheddars, how can I be certain of selecting the best value, the best taste, or exactly the one my wife will like? Being of a moderately obsessional turn of mind, I try to contain my anxiety by doing a mathematical calculation of how many different options there must be here: nationality times maturity, maturity times fat content, fat content times price band, and so on. The arithmetic soon falters. First, it is clear that the grid may have gaps in it (the Welsh seem to make mature vegetarian Cheddar, but the Irish do not). I also start to have serious doubts as to whether I fully understand the taxonomy of Cheddar: is there such a thing as a mild farmhouse or an extra-mature non-vintage? I even begin to wonder if I shall need to invoke Venn diagrams or algorithms to sort the problem out.

Then something else occurs to me. The cheeses are not laid out systematically. Their arrangement is apparently haphazard. Low fat Irish Cheddar jostles alongside Olde Mother Bassington's Superior Special Original Connoisseur Edition from the Cheddar Gorge, but nowhere near any of its creamier compatriots. Expensive cheeses are mixed promiscuously with the cheapos. If you are searching for a mild English vegetarian cheese – and suddenly I remember that is exactly what my wife asked for – you may need to scrutinise the contents of this cabinet for hours.

Finally, I understand. There is method in this madness. I am being bamboozled for a reason. The proprietors of this supermarket do not want me to make a rational choice. Quite the contrary. The ridiculous volume of information, the gratuitous scale of alternatives, and the brazen attack on my cognitive ability are all calculated to render me incapable of choice. As a result, I will almost certainly end up choosing a cheese impulsively and at random. I will be left, of course, with the feeling that I could have chosen better. Like a teasing lover, the supermarket has promised me all, but will deliver so little that I will surely be coming back for more.

Having got a handle on this, I find that my mind starts to wander to another topic: choice in health care. Perhaps this is not surprising. In British political discourse, the issue of 'choice for patients' has acquired enormous prominence.

Politicians now vie with each other to proclaim that choice is the route to patient autonomy, to increased consumer influence, and therefore to raised standards. At one level, this is entirely welcome. However, the example of the cheese cabinet may indicate what happens when choice alone is king.

What I most longed for when I stood by the cheese counter was for a friend to appear unexpectedly from around the corner to say: 'Go for the own-brand farmhouse, John. It's fantastic!' In much the same spirit, our patients often ask us: 'What would *you* recommend?' or 'What would you do if you were in my shoes?' These questions might appear like passivity, or as attempts to evoke paternalism, but usually they are not. They are forms of acknowledgement that what raises people's fears is the unknown and the overwhelming, and what allays it is trust and human connectedness.

There is, in fact, a certain cynicism about placing such an emphasis on choice. In the real world, as opposed to the virtual one that politicians so often seem to inhabit, many of the neediest people cannot actually exercise very much choice in these matters for all sorts of reasons: infirmity, urgency, distance from other providers, the complexity of their needs, or the natural wish to be near their families. But even for the small proportion of patients who are wealthy and well enough to travel anywhere for their medical care, choice may not be so very liberating either. Giving them a list of the nearest eight hospitals, together with records on surgical mortality, cross-infection and a vast array of other parameters, may only raise their anxiety – for who can ever be sure that they could not have had their gall bladder or cataract removed just a little more slickly, a little more painlessly, somewhere else? Like the bewildering range of produce in the supermarket, vast amounts of information may offer our patients a superficial illusion of perfect control and contentment, but in reality it signifies turning care into commodities, and communities into consumers.

16

LET'S TALK
ABOUT SEX

....

'Do you ever find your patients sexually attractive? Have
you ever been sexually aroused while seeing a patient? Have
you ever prolonged a physical examination because you were
enjoying the sight of someone's body? Have you ever had an
enduring sexual fantasy about one of your patients? Have you
at any time considered initiating a sexual relationship with a
patient?' Over the past year or so, I have become particularly
interested in these questions. I have also become curious about
why it seems impossible for most doctors to discuss them.

In ten years as a GP trainer, for example, I can remember
having only one conversation with one of our trainees about
sexual feelings. He was seeing a patient who was becoming
infatuated with him, and possibly vice versa. I handled the
matter rather awkwardly: I was able to talk about the patient's
feelings and what they might mean, but was too embarrassed
at the time to help the registrar to speak about his. Fortunately,
it all ended well and safely. More recently, I have been running
workshops for medical educators on supervision, and I have
been struck by how even the most experienced groups and
individuals will skirt round the subject of sexual feelings, or
address them with coyness. This happens even when we are
talking about cases where these feelings are patently present.

Why is it that we find it so hard to own up as doctors to our desires as sexual animals? One reason, I suspect, is that we are participants in a far wider social game of denial. Almost every newsagent and garage in the country sells sexually explicit magazines, while the internet has thousands of websites showing nothing but sexual acts. You can find the contact details for sex workers in thousands of phone boxes and shop windows. Yet in spite of this glaring evidence, most of us continue to speak as if masturbation, or paid sex with strangers, were aberrant activities, compared with the assumed norm of satisfied monogamy, with perhaps an affair now and again. There certainly seems to be no measured discussion in society at large about the difficulties of *managing* lust, and the pressures, disappointments and shame that are attendant upon so many people's attempts to do so.

In this respect, I have found conversations with gay friends enlightening. Because of their relatively marginalised status, it seems commoner for gays to share confessions with each other concerning the strength and unmanageability of their sexual urges, and to disclose the stratagems – successful or otherwise – that they have tried out in order to satisfy these. Whether frenziedly promiscuous, celibate or loyal to one partner, they often seem to find it easier to talk to each other about what they are feeling and doing without the double standards or dissimulation that go on in much of the straight world.

I wonder if we could also learn lessons by thinking more calmly about paedophiles and our attitudes towards them. Being predominantly attracted to children is probably no more a conscious choice than being attracted to male or female adults: any kind of sexual orientation is programmed at an early age, whether by life experience or by biology. I suspect that many people with paedophile tendencies manage to sublimate them quite successfully into kindliness or intellectual friendships with children. (I believe that I had several teachers at school of whom this was true.) I have also known some highly responsible parents of both sexes who confessed to being aroused at times by the touch or smell of their own children. Yet there is a widespread belief that people with erotic feelings towards children are automatically evil, and can never manage to suppress these feelings.

This conveniently gets the rest of us off the hook: it implies that 'we' do not really have any problems in managing our sexuality, whereas 'they' all do. And by holding on to this belief, we may be pushing some paedophiles further towards becoming abusers, since we damn them equally whether or not they enact their desires.

Whether or not this is the case, the confusion between desire and enactment may be what stops us talking about such matters more sensibly even as doctors. The confusion seems to be more acute for male doctors. Yet we know that sexual desire can become heightened in many situations, including some medical ones such as deaths and disasters. Counsellors and therapists are used to treating such feelings as data – important information about what is going on in the room, and the kind of information that needs to be discussed frankly. The difficulty we have as doctors in openly discussing our sexual feelings towards patients may lead to unnecessary shame among colleagues who are in fact behaving quite impeccably. It also blinds us to what is being done under our noses and in consultation rooms by a minority of colleagues who do actually molest or rape patients. Desire is not a crime. Sexual abuse – of children, patients or trainees – is. In the work I do with medical educators, I am now trying to be a bit braver in naming sexual feelings and in creating a climate in which they can be discussed.

I suspect that many doctors are dealing at any one time with at least one patient (or colleague or junior) where it might be positively helpful to be able to discuss such issues maturely and in confidence. Personally, I doubt if there is any single doctor, of whatever gender or sexual orientation, who could not give the answer yes to many or most of the questions at the beginning of this article – if this could be done safely. If doctors were able to acknowledge more that we are physical beings who have physical feelings and that, like everyone else, we face a moral struggle to manage these, it might in the end protect patients more than if we stay silent.

17

MYSTERIES OF
THE MALE

....

Why do males exist? If you learned biology at school, your teachers will probably have told you it was because combining genes from different individuals – one male and one female – increases variation in a species, and it is variation that helps a species survive.

Unfortunately, most evolutionary experts stopped believing in this explanation over thirty years ago. From a reproductive point of view, no individual is interested in anything very much beyond donating genes to the next generation. As far as whole species are concerned, they are preserved or wiped out more or less at random, largely according to the whims of climate and geology. In addition, you don't actually need sexes to produce variation: the vast majority of organisms like microbes happily mutate and vary without sex.

The great evolutionist John Maynard Smith regarded sex as more or less inexplicable. He talked of 'the twofold cost of males'. First, it is incomprehensible that any female should want to throw away half her genes and take on someone else's, when theoretically she could just produce clones of herself instead. Secondly, the males of many species are entirely useless at doing anything except sitting around, getting fat at the females' expense, and – in the words of

Richard Dawkins – duffing up other males. Among some animals, such as elephant seals, the vast majority of males die as wasteful, disappointed virgins.

Given this wastefulness, it is perhaps not surprising that there are at least forty species where the female kills the male during or after sex. In the case of the praying mantis, she literally bites his head off as part of foreplay, and he carries on in a delighted reflex of posthumous orgasm. Females of other species are equally imaginative: male scale insects have been demoted to microscopic excrescences on their females' legs, while female angler fish carry their mates on their backs as tiny dwarves.

More pertinently, there are many effective ways of reproducing apart from sex as we understand it. These include simple division and gene exchange. These alone have served bacteria so well that they have produced the longest-enduring of all species on the planet, as well as comprising the greatest number of species, and probably constituting most of the mass of living organisms as well.

Among other organisms, alternative methods of reproduction include budding, hermaphroditism (one individual carrying both kinds of sex organs) and isogamy (two individuals, not distinguished as male and female, combining their genes). There are asexual variants among all sorts of creatures, including jellyfish, dandelions, lichens and lizards. Of the creatures who do reproduce sexually, some species have two sexes, but others have three, or thirteen, or ten thousand, if you are a fungus. Many species alternate between sexual and asexual reproduction, either on a regular basis or occasionally, as the circumstances require. Bdelloid rotifers – tiny invertebrates who live in drains and puddles – went off sex about eighty million years ago, and have cheerfully diversified into several hundred species since then without regaining the inclination. Maynard Smith described them an 'an evolutionary scandal', since they seemed to disprove the assumption that sex was in any way a biological advance.

The various current theories about why males evolved and still remain in existence are nicely set out in Matt Ridley's book *The Red Queen*. They are also covered in Olivia Judson's racy and wonderfully informative volume, *Dr Tatiana's Sex Advice to All Creation*. Different theories rejoice in names like Muller's ratchet, Kondrashov's hatchet, and the eponymous Red Queen of Ridley's book (named after the Lewis Carroll character in *Through the Looking-Glass* who perpetually runs without getting very far because the landscape moves with her). This last theory seems to be the front runner at the moment. It is based on the idea that sex is part of a continual race to outwit germs.

What is clear, however, is that the consensus that existed on this topic from Darwin until around the 1980s has totally broken down. The purpose of males has instead become one of the biggest unanswered questions in science. My guess is that we will eventually come to understand fertilisation by males as an evolutionary compromise, poised half way between invasion and alliance, parasitism and symbiosis, or genetic rape and informed consent. There is already much evidence to show how females resist the process biologically (for example by stripping male sperm of part of their DNA) and how males try to control reproduction against their females' will (for example, by killing off competitor sperm in the female genital tract, or alternatively killing the competitors and their offspring directly later on).

If the purpose of males in evolutionary terms is equivocal, the consequences of having two sexes are not reassuring for males either. In a review of the evidence relating to human males, my colleague and mentor Sebastian Kraemer has set out the scale of the problem. Throughout life, men are more vulnerable than women on most measures. This starts with the biological fragility of the male foetus, leading to 'a greater risk of death or damage from almost all the obstetric catastrophes that can happen before birth'. If they survive these catastrophes, boys then have a far greater susceptibility to developmental disorders than girls. These are magnified in turn by our cultural assumptions about masculinity, and by our low expectations of males. The toxic interaction of biological and social ingredients shows itself in far higher rates of suicide and deaths through violent crime.

Males also do worse in (among other things) scholastic achievement, emotional literacy, alcoholism, substance abuse, circulatory disorders, diabetes, and longevity. Kraemer looks at how male disadvantage is 'wired in' from infancy and persists to the grave, but he suggests that we shouldn't necessarily conclude that maleness is a genetic disorder. Instead, he argues, we should show more curiosity about the reasons for boys and men being so vulnerable, and should pay more attention to redressing this in child-rearing and in medicine. Although Kraemer does not mention this, it is also reasonable to speculate that patriarchal societies are, ironically, men's' way of trying to assert their own needs in the face of their patent inferiority.

It may be no coincidence that questions about the *raison d'être* for males, and concerns about their relative deficiencies, should have arisen at this point in history; enough of the relevant information would probably have been available to an observer in Darwin's time. The recent appearance of these scientific preoccupations may well be the consequence of understandable male anxiety. In the last few generations of our species, female control over fertility has developed at a rate so phenomenal that it may justify comparison with the sudden emergence of male-female reproduction itself, around a thousand million years ago. In evolutionary terms, it has taken only the twinkling of an eye from the introduction of the vaginal diaphragm and the contraceptive pill in the middle of the last century, to the widespread use of frozen sperm and extracted eggs, and hence the actualisation of human egg cloning. Within the span of just one lifetime, women have advanced through several enormous stages of biological liberation, and have reached the threshold of virgin births.

Assuming that the minor technical problems of gene damage during cloning can soon be overcome, and that legal constraints will in time be removed – assumptions that seem reasonable by any standard – it is possible that the women of our species will soon have the overall choice of doing with very few men, or with none at all. If, in the mean time, they can prevent males from destroying the planet as a viable habitat for humans, they might be forgiven if they choose to follow the path that has already been pioneered by the bdelloid rotifers. Attempts to understand maleness or to redress its difficulties will then become entirely academic.

18

THE ENDURING
ASYLUM

....

'Loonies,' they shouted from the back of the coach. 'Loonies!' I can't remember if we had reached the gates of the mental hospital yet, but I was excruciatingly embarrassed, and I prayed that they would stop. It didn't help me very much that I understood, to an extent, what had provoked some of the students in my year to such cruel mockery. It was 1974. Sociology had just become a compulsory subject at our medical school in London. The young sociology lecturers had arrived with a mission to radicalise the next generation of doctors, offering us the latest critiques of medicine and of psychiatry. An instructive coach trip into the countryside, to visit one of the vast Victorian 'bins' that still peppered Hertfordshire, Essex and Surrey, was not proving to be helpful.

In retrospect, we were all caught up a painful historical drama concerning views of madness. The sociologists were fired with a conviction that everything we were about to see in the mental asylum was a demonstration of how society oppressed and imprisoned free spirits in the name of medical treatment. The students felt provoked by this, and were no doubt fearful as well, and they regressed into viciousness. While our tour leaders looked forward to a Utopia in which schizophrenics would all be revealed as artists and mystics, the young men on the back seat were imitating the visitors who went to gawp and jeer at the inmates of Bedlam three centuries earlier.

I remember little of the rest of the visit. It is possible that the lecturers cut it short in order to pre-empt a scandal. But I do remember a visit some time later to another rural asylum, for the mentally handicapped, where dozens of adult men just sat in chairs and rocked, or wandered aimlessly around the room, in a way that seemed more like a parody of imbecility than a demonstration of it. Then, during my clinical years, I was sent for about four weeks to study at another, different 'bin' for the mentally ill. Politicians had already decided to shut down all the psychiatric hospitals, but at this stage most of them were still much the same as a century before.

In the place I was assigned to, the corridors were allegedly the longest in Europe. On some of the chronic wards, scores of elderly women sat quite passively, staring into the air; it was said that some of them had been admitted decades earlier for having had illegitimate children. In the acute wards, one could still encounter the 'classic' cases described in the textbooks: people with agitated depression wringing their hands all day long, patients in a state of catatonia sitting like pale statues cemented into place, and psychotic individuals babbling 'word salad'. A hundred years after the French neurologist Charcot showed off his 'hysterics' to visiting colleagues, and more than a decade after R.D. Laing's scathing exposure of such spectacles, ward rounds still consisted of patients appearing every week or two in front of a panel of doctors and psychiatric nurses to 'display' their pathology.

It is now more than a generation later. These memories were stirred up by attending a coffee morning to mark the launch of a book telling the history of the North Wales Hospital. Like the great asylums around London, the hospital once housed fifteen hundred mental patients and employed around a thousand staff. Since its closure in 1995, the grand buildings have stood empty, decaying quietly while developers and councils wrangle over their future. The town's identity has been stamped with its ambiguous inheritance as a centre of care and of incarceration. In some ways it is still waiting to find a new purpose as a community, when these wrangles are resolved.

At the book launch, two former psychiatric nurses from the hospital (one now a historian, and author of the book) mourn the passing of the institution, but with no illusions or regrets. They are reconciled to the harm that it did, both to its inmates and to themselves. Now in retirement, they work for voluntary organisations, visiting some of the people who were discharged from the wards into homes around the town, and making sure that their everyday needs are being met. Ironically, they explain how they now feel discounted as mere volunteers by the professionals who populate the brave new world of community mental health care. For example, psychiatric reports are written with no mention of their work with patients, or of the social activities they lay on to keep these people's minds alive.

Listening to them, I am reminded of how we still remain influenced by the asylum mentality. The asylums of brick and stone, thank God, have now been closed down; we have learned to acknowledge that the madness we observed there was largely manufactured by the institutions themselves, rather than in the minds of their inhabitants. But the virtual asylums have endured. As the two nurses have discovered, we remain in a state of mind where professionals can still ignore any involvement from carers. There is also the mental health 'team', where anonymity and bureaucracy stand in place of the former iron gates and locked wards. We construct another asylum out of the self-important distinctions by which a dozen different mental health professions and theoretical camps insist on identifying themselves and bewildering everyone else. Finally, there are the tick-box inventories by which we try to pretend that mental distress can be reduced to the same kind of diagnostic categories as TB or appendicitis, and entirely divorced from any social or cultural context.

The foolish boys shouting 'Loonies' on the bus to Shenley could never have dreamed that the whole site would one day be converted into luxury homes for City commuters and the rural rich, as it is now. I hope that today's medical students will see a day when our own virtual asylums vanish, and are replaced in their turn by more humane care.

19

DO NOT DISTURB

....

The waiting room was clean and tidy but rather drab, and lacking in any friendly touches such as paintings or historical photos. What particularly caught my attention were the notices on the walls and around the reception desk. 'Don't consume food and drink, or chew gum in the waiting room.' 'Don't ask the doctors for housing letters as we do not issue them.' 'Unused drugs cost the NHS £5.2 billion pounds a year' (how does anyone know, I wondered) 'so don't ask for items that you don't really need.' 'Remember that appointment slots are only for ten minutes. Don't compromise your care by asking the doctor to deal with more than one problem.' Altogether, I counted eleven 'don'ts' and not one 'please'.

I was only there to interview one of the doctors, not as a patient, but I felt quite desolate nonetheless. I pondered on the peculiar idea that medical problems should all be presented singly. Would you be allowed to mention, for example, that you had both chest pain *and* shortness of breath? If you were worried about a sore throat, would the worry disqualify you from mentioning the throat, or possibly vice versa? I recalled a patient I once saw who came in and said, 'I've got three problems.' Acting on an intuition, I asked her, 'What's the fourth?' She told me. It was the problem that she both dreaded and desperately wanted to tell me, and we never got back to the original three problems. I considered telling this anecdote to the doctor once he called me through, and perhaps to talk a little about making space for narratives in medicine as well as numbers. But I was here to conduct research, not to deliver a homily, so I dismissed the idea from my mind.

A receptionist led me upstairs. This was clearly not a doctor used to coming to greet colleagues, let alone patients. He did at least stand up to shake my hand: a smart, pleasant, efficient-looking young man. After some social niceties, I took him through the preliminary part of the interview, which addressed various ethical dilemmas that GPs face in their everyday work. He was thoughtful about them, to a degree, but took little time to reach a clear conclusion on each. Every time he did so, there was a distinct tone of finality in his voice. I had no difficulty imagining what it would be like to be a patient of his. If my blood pressure was high, for example, every ounce of his authority would be harnessed to persuading me to swallow the optimal medication. But if I wanted to speak of matters of the heart, or of the soul, I would have no expectation of being heard, and would keep them to myself.

As part of the research, I asked him if he could give me an example of one recent ethical dilemma that he had handled well, and another where he had doubts about what he had done. In response, he mentioned two encounters that he felt had both gone rather well. In the first, he had to explain to a childless woman of forty that there was no funding available locally for someone of her age to have IVF. The second patient was a community nurse, a few years away from retirement, who was seeing him regularly with minor illnesses in order to request sick certificates. He seemed proud of having told her the previous day that enough was enough, and she should now return to work. He told these stories in a clipped, peremptory manner. I did not get any impression that he had tried to engage with the painful existential struggles that presumably lay under the surface of these requests. I took the risk of mentioning to the doctor that he seemed unperturbed, and possibly imperturbable, by any of these dilemmas. I inquired what perturbed him in his everyday life outside medicine. To do him justice, he blushed slightly and told me about an incident when he got angry with one of his children. But when I asked if such anger ever played a part in his consultations he looked perplexed, and I knew I could not go there.

Doctors like this have a strange effect on me. I start to become anxious that my pre-occupation as an educator with such things as dilemmas, narratives, feelings, ethics, complexity, meaning and consultation skills is really just a projection of my own tortured psyche. Maybe if my upbringing had not been troubled, or if I had not had any therapy, or trained as a therapist, I would see the world in its true light, just as this man sees it: in terms of right and wrong, black and white, and problems that come only in the singular and never in the plural. I begin to wonder if I really am a doctor, or if I have ever been one. I certainly feel at moments like this that I have never been a very skilled or knowledgeable one. Perhaps I have just muddled through in a fog of doubts and uncertainty, never actually making anyone better – unless this was going to happen anyway.

In this state of mind, I closed the interview and made my exit, but as soon as I was back in the waiting room I saw all those 'don'ts' again and my sense of self returned. So too did my sense of the impoverishment of this man's experience of medicine. For what notices like this in waiting rooms really proclaim is this: 'We are afraid. Afraid of intimacy, afraid of suffering, afraid of everything we do not understand and cannot cure.' And the missing 'pleases' are all too clear as well: 'Please remember that you are here to make doctors feel good about ourselves, not the other way around. Please do not challenge us because, in reality, we simply could not cope if you did.'

20

BURNING YOUR
RELATIVES

If you want to dispose of a dead body, either human or animal, there are only a few ways you can do it, and they all have much the same effect. You can leave the body out in the open, so that other creatures of various kinds can eat most of it, metabolising it into water and carbon dioxide. The bits that remain will be oxidised, essentially undergoing the same process but more slowly. An alternative option is to burn the body. This will also lead to the same results, but of course at a much faster rate. Or you can slow the process down by burying the body in the earth or at sea. In that case, consumption of the body by other creatures may still take place, but oxidisation of the uneaten remains will not occur until the body is somehow exposed to the atmosphere once more.

In certain circumstances, geological change on top of a burial site will compress bodies and reposition them at increasing depths under the surface of the earth; in the case of some species – marine animals are a case in point – they may remain there for considerable periods of time, perhaps even millions of years. If you eventually disinter such long-buried corpses in the form of their liquefied or gaseous residues, you can ignite them with a spark in an enclosed space, and produce a very accelerated form of combustion, thereby releasing great amounts of energy. This process was perfected around 150 years ago, when Etienne Lenoir invented the internal combustion engine. Since then, we have been burning dead plankton at a tremendous pace. At a rough estimate, reserves of marine corpses took about a hundred million years to build up (although in reality this probably took place only in short epochs during that time). We have probably got through over half of these reserves already, and at the present rate of usage the rest is unlikely to last us more than another few generations. Currently we are burning dead marine animals at around a million times the rate that it took to create them. This is comparable to raising a fellow human being for twenty-five years and then burning them up for fuel purposes alone in around a minute.

There are a number of peculiarities about this business. One is that we are undoing a planetary process that has allowed us to emerge as a species, and to survive. If every organism remained on the surface of the earth after death, decomposition would soon replace much of the oxygen in the atmosphere with carbon dioxide. This would possibly reduce the net balance of surviving animals to nil. It is only the accidental burial of a large proportion of creatures that has sustained enough free oxygen to result in our own existence, and we are now reversing that process. Another peculiarity is our emotional disengagement from what is happening. Even if we are aware of the fact intellectually, we do not as a rule drive around in our cars exclaiming: 'Oh my God, I am cremating my ancestors and cousins in prodigious quantities, and turning them into noxious gases!' But that of course is exactly what we are doing.

It has become fashionable recently to try to become aware of some of the damage that we are doing by burning our fossils, not because we are worried about oxygen depletion in the very long term but because it will warm up the globe in the very short term. There are now schemes that allow you to calculate how much carbon dioxide you are putting into the atmosphere personally, mainly through the means of transport that you use, and to 'pay it back' symbolically by funding the planting of trees. These schemes are based on units of carbon consumption per year, although an alternative approach would be to look instead at the time it took to create the fuel we consume, and to compare this with the time it takes us individually to burn it up. It seems that the planet produced around 380 thousand billion litres of oil in total; according to this estimate, a three-hour car trip up the motorway using 38 litres of fuel will consume roughly the amount that it would have taken the entire earth five minutes to produce. On this basis, it should be fairly easy to work out how many 'earth hours' of fossil production you use up each year by car travel. (I have done the sums on the back of the proverbial envelope, since I cannot find these calculations anywhere else. Even if my arithmetic is out by some orders of magnitude, I doubt if the result would be reassuring.)

One irony about this rate of oil consumption is that we are using the stuff up so fast that it may run out before the effects of its combustion become terminal. Economists and politicians tend to speak out either about global warming, or about the exhaustion of oil supplies, but they rarely address both at the same time. Yet the real challenges that face the world are likely to be due to the social and political consequences of a coincidental interplay between these two processes. There is no logical reason why global warming should not have happened long before we were able to use up all the oil, or vice versa, and it is tempting to imagine some unfathomable meaning in the fact that these are more or less going to converge. In reality, it may simply depend on how fast we oxidise what is left of our marine ancestors, and whether we finish doing so before their combustion products have the effect of extinguishing ourselves.

21

THE PROBLEM
WITH SEX

....

It is 29 November 1911. In a hired lecture hall, the Vienna
Psychoanalytic Society is holding its regular weekly meeting.
As usual, Professor Freud is in the chair. He has a great deal
on his mind. His movement is splitting into factions. Last
month, he had to expel a group of dissidents – the followers
of Alfred Adler – for placing too much emphasis on the role
of biology in mental illness. The previous day, one of the
most eminent psychiatrists in Europe, Eugen Bleuler, sent
him a resignation letter, arguing that dogmas and expulsions
were more appropriate for a cult or a political party than the
advancement of science. Storm clouds are gathering too in
Freud's relationship with his own chief disciple, Carl Jung.
Their disagreement is not about biology, but about the place
of religion and mythology in understanding mental illness.
Things are not looking good, and possibly the movement may
not survive. The speaker that evening, a young Russian Jewish
woman, is a new member and has just qualified as a doctor.
Probably, Freud has invited her to speak in order to try to
build bridges with Jung.

The young woman in question, Sabina Spielrein, had
an unusually close connection with Jung, being in quick
succession his patient, research assistant, student and lover.

When she was a teenager, she appears to have had a severe bereavement reaction to the death of her only sister from typhoid. This included depression, hysterical behaviour and manic rages. Her parents sent her from Rostov-on-Don in southern Russia to Switzerland, where she ending up in the care of Jung. Using a mixture of word association techniques and very rudimentary psychoanalysis, Jung elicited her private obsessions with beatings and masturbation. He encouraged her to work with him in his psychological laboratory, partly as a kind of occupational therapy. The following year she entered medical school. She then had a sexual relationship with Jung, who was ten years her senior and already married.

Freud knew all about this, as Jung had sought Freud's advice about managing her strong emotional attachment to him, and after some evasion had eventually confessed the degree of his involvement with her. Freud had been indulgent. 'In view of the kind of matter we work with,' he wrote to Jung, 'it will never be possible to avoid little laboratory explosions.' When it became clear that Jung's affair with Spielrein was untenable, Freud mediated between them – again by letter, and somewhat disingenuously – to avert a scandal.

There was nothing surprising in any of this. In the early days of psychoanalysis, there was a determined opposition to any form of sexual hypocrisy, and at times the boundaries of treatment became unclear. Several of the other early analysts had sexual relations with patients. Some patients later came to see their initiation into the psychoanalytic world through both verbal and carnal intercourse as abuse. Others, like Spielrein, experienced it as liberating. The analysts concerned, all doctors, seem to have avoided any legal or professional sanctions. Freud would also have been unperturbed by Spielrein's psychiatric history. As historians have argued, the dramatic way that intelligent young women presented themselves to doctors at that time was largely due to the oppressive social and family circumstances in which they had to live. In the hands of psychoanalysis, they sometimes recovered with miraculous speed, in part because their analysts simply spent time listening to them and validated their frustrations and their sexual desires. Freud's early circle also resembled in some ways a modern self-help group. Its members shared their private lunacies and lusts openly with each other, in lectures, letters, and thinly disguised case histories. One reads these disclosures with both shock and admiration. If we no longer share confessions of our own inner turmoil with each other in this way, it may be because we have learned how explosive this can be – but it may also be through a loss of courage.

All of this may be fascinating, but it is less fascinating than what the young Sabina Spielrein argued in her presentation on that Wednesday night in Vienna. She raised the question of why sexual desire gives rise to pleasure, but also to fear and disgust. 'One feels the enemy inside oneself, in one's glowing love which forces one, with iron necessity, to do what one doesn't want to do: one feels the end, the fleetingness, from which one vainly tries to flee…' In order to make sense of this contradiction, Spielrein proposed that every human being is fated to manage a conflict between two fundamental instincts. On the one hand, there is a wish to survive and prosper as an individual: something that requires independence. On the other hand, there is an evolutionary drive towards reproduction, where the self is dissolved in another person, and death is foreseen. Having presented her thesis in terms of biology and psychology, Spielrein elaborated it with references to literature and mythology – including Tristan and Isolde, Adam and Eve, and tales from the Talmud, where sex and death are symbolically intertwined.

What Spielrein had presented was truly audacious. In the words of one of her biographers, it had 'all the elegance of a new theorem in mathematics or physics'. She had also understood, with remarkable clarity, that psychoanalysis would only make sense if it could be aligned with the theory of evolution. Sadly, Freud's response to the 'little girl' (in his words) was dismissive. He clearly cared little for her biological theory, and criticised her reliance on mythology. 'I must say she is rather nice and I am beginning to understand,' he subsequently wrote to Jung, with what sounds like a laddish wink. 'What troubles me most is that Miss Spielrein wants to subordinate the psychological material to biological criteria…' Psychoanalysis, in Freud's view, had to constitute a science of its own, and not depend on any other field of knowledge.

Six months afterwards, Spielrein moved to Berlin, away from both Freud and Jung, although (almost uniquely) she remained on good terms with both of them. She continued to address conferences and to publish her ideas. Ironically, both Freud and Jung used and adapted some of these ideas in their later writings, but without the emphasis on biology, and with only a grudging acknowledgement to her. In Spielrein's subsequent career, she worked with some of the greatest names in the history of twentieth-century psychology and neuroscience. In Geneva, she collaborated with – and psychoanalysed – Jean Piaget, one of the towering figures of the century in developmental psychology. After she returned to Russia in 1922, she worked with two other seminal thinkers, A.R. Luria and Lev Vygostsky. Unlike her three brothers, she managed to survive Stalin's purges. However, in 1941 the German army occupied Rostov-on-Don. Spielrein and her two daughters, along with the entire Jewish population of the city, were rounded up and summarily shot.

There are many lessons to draw from Sabina Spielrein's extraordinary life. A variety of people have done so in books, on film and on the stage. My own view is that we have hardly begun to appreciate the importance of her ideas. Her attempts to reconcile psychoanalysis with evolutionary theory and developmental psychology were far ahead of her time. Few in the West saw the need to do so until John Bowlby in the 1950s and 60s. More significantly, Spielrein's ideas about sex are in keeping with much that we have discovered in the last twenty years about the biology of reproduction. As she speculated almost a hundred years ago, there is an irreconcilable tension in biology between the needs of the ego (the 'I') and the needs of our genes to replicate themselves. This may have profound implications for our happiness or unhappiness as human beings. In proposing such an idea, the 'little girl' may have been one of the most far-sighted thinkers of the early twentieth century.

Postscript: Following this article, I wrote a full-length biography of Sabina Spielrein, published in 2014: Launer, J., *Sex Versus Survival: The Life and Ideas of Sabina Spielrein* (London and New York: Duckworth Overlook).

22

THE ART OF
QUESTIONING

....

A physician once saved my life with a question, or more precisely, with two questions.

I had been short of breath for several months. Because I had had some cardiac problems in the past, I called my cardiologist. He thought it sounded like a slight worsening of my mild asthma, and reassured me. As the weeks passed, I had good days and bad, and sometimes I worried more and sometimes less. At some point I organised a chest X-ray and an electro-cardiogram for myself, and I also saw my GP. The tests were normal, there were no physical signs of anything, and the message was one of unconcerned uncertainty. Then one day I could not walk to the shops at the end of the road without stopping. My wife thought that my lips were now slightly blue. She insisted that my GP should send me to hospital.

In the back of my mind I had a nagging fear that I was having pulmonary emboli – clots on my lungs. In any logical sense, this seemed absurd. I had none of the classic symptoms of this, such as pain in my chest or legs, or coughing up blood. I was generally fit, and had not gone on any long flights that year that might have caused such clots. But my mother had died of a pulmonary embolus during a hospital admission. Also, for the first time in my life, I was unaccountably having dreams about her brother, who was murdered by the Nazis as a teenager – almost certainly by cyanide asphyxiation in Auschwitz. I had not known him, and she had virtually never talked about him.

I saw a chest physician who could not have been more thorough, but it was clear from her questions that pulmonary emboli did not figure remotely in her thinking. All the same, when she had finished examining me, she asked, 'Have you come up with any diagnosis yourself?' Sheepishly, and with the slight fear of ridicule that comes with not being a specialist, I told her of my specific anxiety. She then asked one further question, 'Does that mean you'd like a lung scan to reassure you?' I said yes. Three days later it was done, and showed I had already lost twenty-five per cent of my lungs to clots. 'You're a very good diagnostician,' she said, graciously. I never told her about the bad dreams.

At medical school, we are taught meticulously about the importance of asking the right questions. Yet in our subsequent careers we often forget two of the most crucial ones: 'What do you think you've got?' and 'What would you like me to do?' As my physician demonstrated, the art of questioning clearly needs to go beyond the dry litany of formal history-taking and should embrace the patient's view as well. When we remember this, we nearly always save our patients many sleepless nights, and sometimes we save their lives too.

The art of questioning may go further still. One of the most challenging researchers ever to have looked at questions in consultations is the Canadian psychiatrist Karl Tomm. He talks of conversations between professionals and patients as being treatments in themselves. He doesn't mean this in the relatively banal sense of offering reassurance or empathy.

Instead he talks about 'questions as interventions'. He suggests that the chief purpose of clinical questioning is not primarily to pin problems down, but to try and redefine and resolve them through the conversational process itself. As a result of his researches, Tomm has proposed ways of using questions in order to call forth new and unexpected expressions, memories and ideas from the patient, including ones that they might otherwise not have expressed, or even thought. Although Tomm is writing principally about consultations in mental health clinics, his approach to questioning may have equal application to medical contexts. One way of describing the kind of clinical interview that he recommends is as 'conversations inviting change' – a term I have adopted to describe the approach to consultation skills I mainly teach.

Tomm's original paper on questions has a stupefyingly off-putting title and it appears in a journal that few doctors will have heard of. Nevertheless, I would say that it has influenced my professional behaviour more than anything I have ever read – and almost as much as the two questions my chest physician asked that saved my life.

23

HOT WATER

....

When our children were smaller, we once took a family holiday in a Greek beach resort, where doctors seemed to spring out from behind every bush. Counting myself, there were at least seven in the hotel, all British: three GPs, a sexual health physician, an orthopaedic surgeon, a cardiologist and a palliative care specialist. Between us, we could have covered most medical eventualities, and it would have been entertaining to imagine a scenario that might have called for each of our particular skills in turn. Fortunately, it meant that my services as a generalist were only called upon for the less alarming kinds of incident. I removed a speck of paint from the eye of another British tourist whose gratitude was hugely disproportionate. I attended a small girl with a cut on her scalp sustained from a close encounter with a swing. And I advised a number of people who had gone down with gastroenteritis. In fact, an increasing number of guests seemed to be getting gastroenteritis as the fortnight went on. I got it myself for a day. So did two other members of my family.

It was only a few days before the end of the holiday that I considered there might be a connection between these illnesses and something else that I had noticed: there was no hot water in the toilets of the hotel restaurant. I had spoken twice to the reception staff about this quite early in the holiday. They had made appropriate noises of concern, and they reassured me that it would be sorted out – but nothing changed. Once I started to worry about the possible link with so many stomach upsets, I wondered if I should see the manager in person to express my concern. I even thought of suggesting that he should close down the restaurant toilets and ask people to use the ones in their rooms instead, where the water was piping hot. However, I kept putting it off, and in the end I just filled in the hotel feedback form when we left, pointing out the possible reason that so many people had gone down with diarrhoea and vomiting.

After returning home, I was embarrassed to think that I did so little to protest. I also wondered why several of my professional colleagues – some of whom said they had also noticed the lack of hot water – did not complain more forcefully either. The restaurant was a buffet, which meant that everyone used the same serving implements. Transmission of faecal germs must have been happening all the time. I have been trying to work out what led all of us to say nothing about such an obvious health risk.

The most important factor, beyond a doubt, is that we were all having a jolly good time and everything else seemed to be going very smoothly. The seaside setting, surrounded by mountains and overlooking the Ionian Sea, was idyllic. The staff were wonderfully attentive, and they treated all our children like dignitaries rather than detritus (one of the main reasons, apart from the weather, for taking holidays in Mediterranean countries). If there had been many other problems, I am sure that I or one of my colleagues would have managed to harness our dissatisfaction with the lack of hot water, but the raw material for outrage was simply not there. Like most Britons, probably none of us wanted to upset anybody by making a fuss. Personally, I knew from previous visits to Greece that the plumbing there often leaves much to be desired. I managed to reassure myself that I had no definite evidence that more people were getting ill that one might expect among tourists there.

Everything else was going very smoothly ... none of us wanted to upset anybody by making a fuss ... you can't change something that's generally accepted ... no actual proof of a link ... no definite scientific evidence ... it probably would all have happened anyway ... none of the other doctors seemed very bothered ... it was easier to forget about the problem. Does any of this sound familiar? Of course it does. It is the miserable and unconvincing chorus that attends every single health service scandal that ever occurs. What I and my colleagues had enacted on our holidays, with characteristic professional insouciance, was classic medical bystander behaviour. We had played our traditional parts in a simulation of the prologue to systemic disaster, the sort of disaster that befalls the health service time and again, year after year.

It did not feel like that at the time. It felt, of course, like normality. Better than normality, positively hunky-dory. But that precisely is the problem. Apathy is a retrospective diagnosis. If there had been a serious epidemic of gastroenteritis ending in hospitalisations and a catastrophic end to people's summer break, I am sure that we would have reframed the experience very differently. What seemed at first like an idyllic holiday would have been recollected as a nightmare, and our inaction would have become a cause of deep guilt and shame. Next time, I have promised myself, I will make a fuss.

24

INTERPRETING
ILLNESS

....

The first piece of research I ever did was a study of interpreters. I did it on a visit to northern Nigeria as a medical student. I made audiotapes of out-patient consultations between patients who spoke Hausa and doctors who spoke English. I used non-medical staff as interpreters. Once I had made the tapes, I asked some local medical students, all perfectly bilingual, to listen to them and translate all the Hausa statements. I looked at what the patients had actually said and then compared this with what was transmitted by the interpreters.

Not surprisingly, I found all sorts of deviations between the patients' utterances and what the interpreters conveyed. Some of these deviations were quite legitimate. For example, skilled staff could run through part of a medical history on their own initiative and then report, quite accurately: 'His urine's normal' or 'He doesn't have any breathing problems'. On the other hand, I discovered some alarming errors, where interpreters had reported that the patients had said something they had not. Also, the interpreters were pretty selective in what they wanted the doctor to know, and occasionally they even berated patients for what they considered to be vagueness or inconsistencies.

I wrote some guidelines for using interpreters, based on what I found. They went as follows (please excuse the sexist language – it was the 1970s): 'Greet the patient to establish direct contact. Be seen to be in charge of the interpreter. Assess the interpreter's English and try to find out how well he speaks the patient's language. Assess his interests: he may be an anxious relative or an indifferent auxiliary. Give only short sentences for translation, and get the interpreter to explain that the patient must do the same. Make sure everything is translated. Check every answer by asking questions in two or three ways. Finally, use the interpreter to tell the patient everything you would tell him if he could speak your language.'

Forty years later, I would stand by a few of these rubrics, especially the first and last. But I would recant most of the others. Through experience of using interpreters a great deal myself, I have lost my conviction in what one might call the more obsessive, even dictatorial parts of this guidance. Nowadays I believe that the presence of an interpreter, whether in person or by phone link, radically changes the nature of a medical encounter, so that it may be an error to try to force it to resemble something it is not – a one-to-one conversation in a single language. I have even come to think that using interpreters may teach us something important about the nature of all medical encounters and how to conduct them.

I have noticed, for example, that patients speaking in their own language do not like to have their narrative flow interrupted for translation, even when the doctor believes that this needs to happen for diagnostic reasons. To put it at its simplest, it appears that patients want quite literally to be heard, and they may care relatively little whether the main hearer is someone with medical skills or not. I have also noticed that most interpreters, whether they are close relatives of the patient or paid professionals, have personal resources that go beyond the skill of literal, word-for-word, translation. They usually bring to the conversation a wealth of shared cultural associations, and an ability to contextualise utterances that might otherwise be meaningless. Such resources, of course, disprove the notion that 'pure' translation actually exists – an idea that no professional literary translator would ever hold.

As I have become aware of these things, I have increasingly tried to sit back and watch with respect as apparently effective consultations unfold between patient and interpreter in spite of – or because of – my passivity. I am content to understand very little for several minutes at a time, if it looks as if the patient is happy with me doing this. I do this particularly with interpreters whom I have used on many occasions before, and know will alert me if anything worries them from a medical point of view. I take the risk of believing that the exchange is serving the purpose that the patient needs, and I try to suppress a wish to intrude my own professional purposes instead.

I suspect that many of my medical colleagues would feel very uncomfortable with this confession. Equally, I have no doubt that many anthropologists and sociologists would approve. Much contemporary social science research shows how doctors are naïve when they imagine that patients tell us their histories only so that we can formulate an accurate diagnosis or recommend a treatment. These are usually our main preoccupations as doctors, but they may not be the patient's. Illness narratives serve far more urgent and essential purposes. For example, they allow patients, through the very act of speaking, to fashion their memories and sensations into a coherent shape. They provide people with opportunities to assign causation, purpose and direction to their experiences, and to claim moral legitimacy for their own actions. Like all personal narratives, they enable people to describe who they are, to discover who they are becoming, and to define who they wish to be.

Telling a story to another person about one's experiences is a way of locating the self, perhaps even of constructing it. For such a task, it may be that an interpreter is at least as good a collaborator as a doctor, and may be considerably better. Perhaps we should all have interpreters present when we visit our doctors.

25

IT TAKES TWO

....

Over the years, I have spent quite a lot of time thinking, teaching and writing about supervision in medicine. Like most people who have been drawn towards the subject, I have become fascinated by the way that supervision lies at the intersection of factual knowledge and self-awareness, and by the opportunities it offers for both technical and ethical development.

The word 'supervision', I have found, is not at all straightforward. If you move among people like counsellors and psychologists, for example, you will hear them use the word constantly and fairly casually. '*I must get some supervision on a tricky case that I'm seeing*', they say, or '*I'm feeling a bit stuck – would you mind giving me a bit of supervision later?*' They may be asking for an extended conversation about a case, but equally they may be wanting no more than five minutes' chat over lunch. Used in this way, the word seems to carry no special sense of hierarchy or of being judgemental, and no particular sense of formality either. Basically, supervision here means a bit of reflective time, of whatever length, to open up to new ideas.

Doctors, by contrast, often seem rather allergic to the word. Until recently, we tended to avoid the term altogether as a profession, except during training. Even now, many of my colleagues tell me that the idea of getting any kind of supervision as an established professional smacks to them of something bossy and critical, and of telling people how to do their jobs – like a manager standing over someone at a supermarket till. This state of affairs is of course changing, and medics are now beginning to think of supervision in a similar way to other professions: not as having someone looking over your shoulder but as having someone looking after you. Nevertheless, my experience of teaching supervision to doctors is that, even when they manage to shake off their worries about being bossed about, they still think of supervision in terms of being given the 'right answers' to any problem rather than being invited to think about their work in an entirely different way.

What I have learned from mental health professionals – and now attempt to teach to doctors – is that supervision is not a teaching technique but essentially a state of mind where both parties (supervisor and supervised) implicitly recognise the limitations that arise whenever individuals see cases on their own. These limitations can affect us not just in the occasional case that seems to go badly wrong, but also in cases that seem to be going entirely right, but may do so only because we have become too comfortable with the way we do things.

When I see a patient by myself, for example, I am limited not just by the boundaries of my experience and my knowledge base, but also by the fact that I am who I am. I can often make up for the limitations of my experience and knowledge quite easily by using a textbook or the internet, or by knocking on someone's door and asking them a straightforward question. By contrast, the limitations that arise from being myself are inescapable. All the questions I can think of asking the patient, and all the formulations I can think of about the case, simply escape from the inevitable rigidities of the self. Nor will any amount of training ever alter this fact. The only thing that can effectively change my thinking about any case is an encounter with another person who is able to interrogate my certainties, and perturb me into remembering (yet again) that reality always can be seen from many different perspectives.

Seen in this light, the task of supervising another doctor is not principally to explore the gaps in a colleague's knowledge, or to propose alternative actions. It is a more philosophical task: to detect and inquire into any automatic and unexamined habits of thinking and feeling. Whether one is supervising a psychoanalyst or an orthopaedic surgeon, it involves the same fundamental processes: raising a friendly eyebrow at glibness, and interposing a penetrating question into each comfortable elision of thought. Supervision at its best can be deeply disturbing because it leads to each of us being 'found out' – not in the trivial way we may fear, by exposing us as frauds, but in the much deeper sense of discovering how fragile our certainties are.

Supervision should remind us that we are partial and prejudiced human beings, who by preference will nearly always follow the mental and emotional paths we have trodden before, rather than daring to seek new ones. In that sense, giving supervision, and asking for it, may be one of the most truly scientific experiments we ever undertake.

26

YELLOW NOSE SIGN

....

A mother was describing to me how her child had been vomiting over the last few days. 'And I know just before he's going to be sick,' she told me, 'because the sides of his nose turn yellow.' She looked at me significantly, as if she was assuming that the yellow nose sign would mean something to me as a doctor and lead me to the exact diagnosis.

Patients' narratives are full of these kinds of descriptions. Mostly doctors do not even hear them – quite literally. If you watch videos of your own consultations, you find that there are details in every history, mostly about yellow noses and the like, of which you have no recollection. Because they do not fit the medical view of the world, doctors' brains consider them meaningless and they tune out.

The sociologist P.M. Strong pointed out a long time ago that most people are actually caught in a double bind when they see doctors. Often, their main reason for seeing us is precisely because they are not sure if they or their children's experiences fit the patterns of illness that we know about. Yet we doctors get wary if they recite perfect accounts in case they have read them off the internet, and we react with mild contempt when they talk about things we do not understand, like yellow noses.

Social scientists are trained to be more tolerant than doctors. They would take it for granted that the mother genuinely did see her son's nose go yellow each time that he was about to throw up. They would not be troubled by the fact that her notion of yellow did not correspond with my concept of jaundice. They would also be vastly more curious about exploring the beliefs and explanations that enabled her to notice when noses turn yellow. In other words, they would put her perceptions on a level playing field with mine.

What would happen if doctors did this too? One of the books that most influenced me as a medical undergraduate – as it did many other people at the time – was Thomas Kuhn's *The Structure of Scientific Revolutions*. Kuhn argued against the common idea that advances in scientific theory came about as a result of systematic attempts to prove a previous theory wrong. Instead, he proposed a more sociological view. It was one that focused on how people in each generation develop perceptions of the world that do not fit with previous descriptions. Kuhn examined how people generally discount such perceptions at first, assuming that they must be distorted or incorrect because they do not fit with existing theory. Over time, however, more and more people share these perceptions, until they become the nodes around which a new world view starts to coalesce. Once this happens, the old theory simply crumbles away. At first it becomes outmoded, then obsolete, and in time quite incomprehensible.

The best demonstration I know of this process in action appears in an essay about the history of asthma by another sociologist, John Gabbay. He goes through accounts of asthma from the seventeenth century to the twentieth, noting how the shifts from one paradigm to the next are not small evolutionary ones but gigantic philosophical ones. Not only does the knowledge change with each version of asthma, but so does the fundamental nature of that knowledge.

Gabbay points out the temptation to assume that earlier descriptions of asthma will automatically map on to modern descriptions of asthma, or at the very least on to other recognisable conditions like heart failure or cirrhosis. It seems that nothing could be further from the truth. Seventeenth-century asthma does not correspond in any way with modern asthma, but unfortunately it does not remotely correspond with anything else either. People with earlier models of asthma not only believed things we do not believe, but (as Gabbay illustrates in great detail) they saw things we cannot see, used treatments we cannot understand, noticed improvements we cannot believe, and offered explanations that are now totally impossible to follow. Each successive historical version of asthma consisted of a self-referential loop of symptoms, signs, diagnosis and treatment. None of its elements now makes sense to us, or corresponds to anything that can be found in subsequent versions of asthma. The same, Gabbay strongly implies, will eventually be true of our 'asthma' too.

Doctors often find this kind of thinking hard to accept. They believe that twenty-first-century knowledge must be in some way entirely different from *all* previous types of knowledge. They find it hard to accept that even such fundamental notions as anatomy and evidence may one day be replaced by other constructions that we are incapable of even dreaming about. Many sociologists see this limitation in our thinking as simple defensiveness. They would argue that we are locked into our own mindsets first by self-selection as a profession and then by continuing indoctrination. We all feel threatened by the idea that our whole system of scientific belief will one day dissolve. Yet if Gabbay is right, that dissolution is inevitable. And if Kuhn is right, the next medical paradigm may well depend on someone taking yellow noses seriously.

27

DIALOGUE AND DIAGNOSIS

....

This is a story so typical of general practice that you could almost use it to help medical students decide whether or not they want to be GPs. (I have, as always, altered some details in order to make the person involved anonymous.) The patient was a woman in her late thirties, childless. The story had begun about two months before, when I saw her with some peculiar neurological symptoms. I was vaguely aware at the time that she had had a miscarriage about a year previously, but this was not at the front of my mind when I saw her: her immediate symptoms were too worrying to think about anything else.

I called up the duty neurological doctor at the local hospital to describe her symptoms. He thought I was right to worry and offered an urgent out-patient appointment. He saw my patient a week later and was concerned enough to do some scans. These turned out to be entirely normal. When he saw the patient a month afterwards to tell her the results, the symptoms had in any case changed. They had become far less specific and more ones of general muscular fatigue. He sent her back to me with a letter raising the possibility of a chronic fatigue syndrome and suggesting that I should send her to someone with a particular interest in such states.

So I saw her again and went back to square one. This time I got an entirely different story. At this stage, her symptoms were now mainly aches and pains and exhaustion. She had more or less forgotten the numbness and pins and needles that had brought her to me in the first place and caused such concern. (I wonder if they were amplified from the original consultation onwards as a result of seeing doctors, and then dispelled by the normal scans. We sometimes forget that we make our own contribution to the construction of symptoms.) When I asked her to date her problem, she told me this time that she had had them about a year – considerably longer that she had said at first. This timing took us back precisely to her miscarriage.

Miscarriage. Childlessness. Late thirties. Suddenly I knew that I was going to hear quite a different story from the clipped, clinical one that I had elicited, and possibly even promoted, at our previous meeting. And indeed, an entirely new story now came to light. The miscarriage had been, in effect, a cruel caesura in her life. Until she had come to the doctor with heavy bleeding, she told me, she had never even dreamed she might be pregnant. By the time she knew that she was pregnant, it was already over. It was the only pregnancy of her entire life – a much longed-for one that she believed would never happen. But she had lost it before there had been any chance to celebrate her fertility for even one minute.

She began to cry, and then she told me more. Five years previously, when she was still in her mid-thirties, she had gone with her husband for some fertility tests. She was told she needed IVF, but in the same breath the gynaecologist said he could only offer this if she saw him privately –

which she could in no way afford. She described, word for word, the consultation with the gynaecologist. I have heard too many such stories to discount them as exaggerations or misunderstandings. The 'rules' the gynaecologist had invented made no sense, in logic or humanity, but she and her husband clearly had neither the education nor the emotional resources to challenge them. They had walked out of the clinic and never requested or even thought of a second opinion. When she had grieved for her miscarriage a year ago, she had relived every minute of the earlier rebuff, and felt its injustice bitterly. She recognised the cruel pattern in both events: the tantalising possibility of parenthood, coupled instantly with its extinction. Her consequent numbness had not been neurological but existential.

It was clear that she did not have chronic fatigue syndrome and she did not need to see a fatigue specialist. What was evident was that she needed someone to ask for and tolerate a narrative that was entirely different from the one in which we all colluded, perhaps necessarily, the first time round. She also needed to tell someone who was capable of hearing both kinds of story – the biological and the biographical one – and who did not find it at all surprising that human beings live in both worlds at the same time, and may not know which of these worlds to talk about, in order that things might change.

I am sure that encounters like this also happen in hospital and psychiatric out-patient clinics. But as GPs we work permanently on the knife edge, as it were, between the diagnosis of illness and the interpretation of experience. Many GPs have such transforming conversations regularly. And I wonder how on earth one could ever quantify the outcome of these unique exchanges: the time, money and endless frustration that are saved when people are headed off from further referrals, further tests, and further futile 'treatments'; and the healing that may start when a story like this can be told.

28

BREAKING
THE NEWS

....

We all commiserated as our colleague told us about her awful consultation the previous day. She had had to tell a man in his fifties that his ultrasound scan had shown a hard lump in his pancreas, almost certainly cancer. The man clearly hadn't been expecting bad news, and had turned up to the consultation on his own, with a rather jaunty manner. To make matters worse, she had never met the man previously – she was standing in for someone else that day. We squirmed and offered our sympathy as she described the encounter unfolding from moment to moment. She was honest enough to admit that she hadn't actually liked the man, who had been a bit smelly. At the end of the consultation she had wanted to hug him, or at the very least to touch him on the arm, but found herself unable to. We were all experienced medical educators, and we tried to cover every angle in our discussion: the painfully inappropriate circumstances in which we often have to break bad news; the way in which negative impressions can disable our compassion, and how we aspire to the impossible task of spelling out a death sentence nicely, feeling like failures when it never happens that way.

Yet afterwards I pondered on her story and I couldn't get another, heretical thought out of my mind: why did the doctor have to tell the truth? There must have been a dozen ways in which she might have delayed or underplayed telling the man the full scan result, at least until a relative could be present – or until the patient's usual doctor was available. It took little imagination to think of various forms of subterfuge that she might have used: 'the result isn't back yet…', 'it's back but it's not entirely clear…', 'I'm a bit puzzled about its significance and I need to discuss it with a colleague…' If such prevarications had raised the patient's anxiety, would that have been so terrible, especially by comparison with what actually did happen? I recalled that a generation ago, few doctors would ever have dreamed of telling this man the truth in this way. And surely no group of medical educators at that time would have failed to mention, or even to think, that it might have been done differently.

There has been a generational change, but culture makes a difference too. A week after this conversation, I was teaching a group of interpreters mainly from eastern Europe. The same theme arose again. One of them described, with horror, how a friend of hers had been to see a doctor in London who had told him – 'by himself, on the spot, there and then' – that he had cancer of the lymph glands. Back home, she said, no one would ever give someone such information without first checking with the family whether the patient had the resilience to absorb it, or to cope with it. When she said this, her peer group murmured their agreement and expressed their disapproval of the brutal and uncompromising frankness of British doctors.

As it happens, her views find support in cross-cultural research about death and dying. In many parts of the world, and among many cultures, people still take a far more circumspect approach to the disclosure of a terminal illness than we generally do in the West. According to medical anthropologists and family researchers, this may have nothing to do with paternalism or with a fear of being honest. Instead, it may arise from a belief in the crucial importance of sustaining hope as a life force, together with a radically different understanding of the duties of the individual towards the family and vice versa.

'In cultures where the family is the unit of identity and responsibility,' writes Lucy Candib from the University of Massachusetts, 'interdependence is the higher value, not individualism… The patient knows that family is protecting her and that this is what families should do… Non-disclosure is not a matter of lying. Ambiguity may be seen as the most suitable strategy to allow the patient to maintain tranquillity.' Candib also cautions against making simplistic assumptions that everyone from a certain culture will share the same preference for or against knowing the truth. She advises physicians to 'offer the option of truth' when breaking bad news, regardless of where the patient comes from. She suggests using questions such as these: 'Will you want to be making the decisions about your care with the doctors, or do you want your family to be making those decisions?' and 'When we understand what is causing your illness, will you want us to tell you about it, or to talk with your family about it?'

This kind of sensitivity to cultural and individual norms is gaining increasing support among medical ethicists. Following several decades of so-called 'principlist' ethics (based on the four well-known principles of autonomy, non-maleficence, beneficence and justice), an increasing number of writers now seem to be moving towards a more flexible approach known as 'narrative ethics'. One of its central tenets is that every situation is unique and unrepeatable, and cannot be fully captured by appealing to universal principles. Any decision or action is therefore justified in terms of its fit with the individual life story of the patient, and needs to be sought through conversation rather than based on prior notions.

Seen in this light, our colleague's assumption that there was only one right action when faced with the jaunty man with pancreatic cancer might be seen as an example of die-hard principlism. And we may well see the pendulum swinging away from the practice of telling people the truth, the whole truth and nothing but the truth – at least until the timing and context for doing so are entirely right.

29

CAREERS ADVICE

....

The idea of the career patient came to me out of the blue. I was in a team meeting at another local GP practice. I was listening to a case presentation, of a kind that is dismally familiar. The patient was evidently seeing six consultants in the local hospital and a further three in specialist centres in London. She was on over twenty different kinds of medication, including six different kinds of painkillers. In the past two weeks she had attended two emergency departments, and had alarmed the doctors there sufficiently for both of them to have organised urgent scans of her spine. Her GP was fighting a hopeless battle to try to cut down her drugs, encourage all the doctors to communicate effectively with each other and with him, and reduce the financial impact of her behaviour on the National Health Service. As part of this battle, he had just insisted on seeing her on a weekly basis to 'get to grips with her case', as he put it. Needless to say, she was delighted with this proposal. It was at this point in his presentation that I found myself asking the GP why he felt compelled to disrupt this person's highly successful career as a patient. If she was a physicist or an economist, I suggested, her level of commitment to her life's work, and her degree of imagination and intelligence in pursuing it, might surely have earned her a Nobel prize.

I said this in jest, but it was a serious jest. I was hoping to liberate the GP from his mission to rescue the patient from something she clearly had no desire to be rescued from. I was also trying to debunk an unrealistic expectation that I might be able to propose something magical as an invited 'expert' with pretensions to knowing something about clinical supervision. In doing so, I was drawing on a well-established tradition of using paradoxes in the face of perverse systems and insoluble conundrums. Yet the fact is, I genuinely thought it likely that the only feasible option here was damage limitation: not to the NHS budget, and certainly not to the patient, but just in terms of the GP's time, frustration and exhaustion.

Career patients appear to have most or all of the following characteristics. First, they have a tantalising mixture of indisputable physical problems on the one hand, and a collection of vaguer signs and investigative findings on the other. Almost certainly, someone will have failed to diagnose something fairly obvious like an underactive thyroid gland early on in their careers, and they will apologetically slip this into their accounts, so that every subsequent physician will be wary of leaving even the tiniest stone unturned. Although they may have had numerous treatments and operations, both necessary and pointless, they remain intensely loyal to their doctors, especially those who have most conspicuously failed to improve any of their symptoms. Also, their problems usually accrue slowly and in geological layers, rather than appearing as sudden and dramatic eruptions.

Next, career patients usually have a finely tuned awareness of the workings of the health service. In particular, they have an intimate knowledge of its failings, and its tendencies towards fragmentation and dysfunctional communication.

This gives them an ability to provoke and make a mockery out of the inability of most hospitals or local networks to join things up. Although this is done through intuition and with innocence rather than brazen calculation, they succeed in getting doctors to carry out absurd and improbable interventions (like two scans in a fortnight) in preference to picking up the phone and talking to each other.

There is a very large medical literature on various kinds of patients who in some ways overlap with career patients: they are commonly called frequent consulters, heavy service users, 'fat file' patients, heartsink patients and so forth. Much of this literature purports to offer advice about how to work more productively with such people. Suggested tactics include reattributing symptoms to life events rather than physical causes, involving relatives and carers in consultations, and asking doctors to reflect on the their negative feelings about such cases. Although such advice can be helpful at times (although probably not as helpful as its proponents claim), it never seems to work with genuine career patients. Probably they have too much invested in their career to exchange it for an alternative one, however persuasively this is proposed.

The big question in dealing with career patients, I suspect, is whether it is possible to hold on to a genuine sense of respect for them, as opposed to using the label as a cause for disapproval. One reason for respect is that they are not doing something meaningless. Quite the contrary, their pursuit of medical care fills their lives with purpose. They have an occupation that is just as absorbing as many far more respectable ones and may in fact be less of a drain on the public purse than some others, such as opera-singing. In any case, it is possible that we might end up paying even more for the social consequences of making them redundant. However, the most important reason for respecting them is that their profession is in a complementary relationship with ours: they strive to sustain our existence as we do theirs. Like career patients, doctors too can be devoted to the search for simplistic answers to complex and unfathomable human problems. We are, in a sense, co-dependent.

In the end, the only way we may be able to have any impact on career patients is by accepting their right to pursue their life's work freely. Working on this principle, the GP who presented the case I described has now reduced his patient's regular appointments from weekly to bi-monthly intervals, and is issuing repeat prescriptions on demand, except where he feels he is putting himself at risk legally. I sincerely doubt that his withdrawal from co-dependence will make things worse. It is just conceivable that it might make them better.

30

ONLY OBEYING
ORDERS

....

For a few months, one of the teams I worked in was said to be 'overperforming' its service contract. This word is often used by managers in the National Health Service. Overperformance really just means that you have done more work than predicted, so telling people that they have overperformed is a bit like saying that the sun has overperformed because the weather forecast said that it would rain. All the same, we were asked to cut down on our work for the remainder of the financial year. We had to close some cases, knowing that we might need to reopen them once the new financial year started in April. We also had to change the review dates for other patients, in order to make sure that they didn't darken our doorstep again until April had begun. Where two clinicians from different specialities were seeing a case jointly (fairly common in our line of work), we had to explain that only one of us could see them for the time being.

Fortunately – or ludicrously, depending on which way you look at it – all of this only applied to part of our catchment area. People who lived slightly further away, or in some instances on the opposite side of the same road, continued to have no such restrictions. In theory at least, we could even have decided to fill our time by seeing them more often, or with several clinicians in the room twiddling their thumbs and waiting for March to expire.

This phenomenon, and others like it, are now very common in the National Health Service. Broadly speaking, I have noticed three kinds of reaction among my colleagues to these kinds of directives. A few outspoken staff members burst out with indignation or even outrage when one of these measures is announced. It is usually the same people on every occasion, often the ones who seem angry about a lot of things at work anyway. We admire them, but also feel irritated and embarrassed, wondering why they cannot just accept the madness of everyday life in the health service like the rest of us, knuckle under as we do, and get on with their jobs. By contrast, a number of other colleagues seem to buy into the latest managerial demand more or less wholeheartedly each time. While lamenting any temporary difficulties, they are keen to explain to the rest of us the importance of rational planning, workforce efficiency and so on. Things have been unacceptably sloppy in the past, they remind us, and we are paying the necessary price for tightening systems in the right way. We admire these people too – to an extent – but we are also a bit scared of them. If they aren't already in positions of authority, they probably soon will be.

Most of us, to be honest, fall somewhere in between in our reactions. Our sympathies are with the protesters, and we may even make some tame comments to this effect, but nevertheless we fall in with the modernisers. We take their rebuke to heart, as if overperformance isn't just an artefact of budgeting, but a genuine moral failing. And we try to convince ourselves that it isn't as insane as it seems to postpone seeing a referral because it's March and the patient's address is in Jubilee Road and not Jubilee Avenue.

As always, I am struck by how these processes resemble totalitarianism. I realise that some people will find this comparison preposterous, and clearly one has to discriminate between degrees of totalitarianism: there is an important difference between being told off for overperformance and being shot for it. Yet all the classical ingredients are there: the idealisation of order, the marginalisation of dissent, the disqualification of compassion, enthusiastic collaboration by some thoroughly decent citizens, and passivity among the rest of us. There is also a certain kind of collusive secrecy. When we change patients' appointments around, or send letters telling them their files have now been closed, we don't necessarily tell them the real reasons. Instead, we package these in some other convenient form, somewhere along the spectrum from coincidental half-truths ('we have decided to close every case where patients have not attended their last two appointments') to downright lies ('unfortunately Dr Launer is unable to be present at our next meeting'). Without any discussion, we collectively assume that we cannot be open with our patients. The deceit becomes part of the climate in which we work.

In discussing totalitarianism, the historian Hannah Arendt famously wrote of the banality of evil, and it is indeed banality that characterises these sinister incremental shifts in what is acceptable. After the team meeting where we learned about our overperformance, I probably went to the canteen in my usual way, and then took my cappuccino downstairs to my office so that I could dictate the necessary letters. Fairly soon afterwards, I would have more or less forgotten this latest small assault on my capacity to practise professionally, or humanely. My job and my pension were still intact, so perhaps things weren't really so bad after all...

31

THE ART OF NOT
LISTENING

....

One of the most gifted psychologists I ever knew had the knack of going to the heart of the matter in any conversation. This could be irritating at times as it made everyone else feel so plodding. Usually it was impressive, because it saved his patients and colleagues so much wasted time and misplaced emotion. It seemed a knack that was well worth acquiring, but if you asked him how he did it, he said, 'I just tune out a lot.'

It is arresting to think that *not* listening might be a crucial professional skill. During our basic training as doctors, we spend a great deal of time learning how to listen carefully for patterns of description that fit particular diseases. Later, as we develop the art of consulting, we realise how important it is to pick up not just the verbal signals, but the words in between that hint at such things as disappointment, anger, pleading or despair. I spend a great deal of time in my work as an educator in helping experienced doctors notice how much they normally miss, and in training them – through supervision, group work, video analysis or role play – to improve their capacity to pay attention to what patients say. How strange, then, to hear a renowned psychologist disclose the secret of his expertise as 'tuning out'.

The claim makes sense, though, at many levels. In biological terms, for example, we are coupled with our environment so that we only notice those forms of information that affect our survival. (We do not see air, for example, simply because it is always there, so we do not need to be able to recognise a vacuum.) Similarly, in social terms, we are habituated to pick up the cues that matter most in our own milieu, but will miss a huge amount if transposed to unfamiliar settings or cultures where nuances of gesture that we do not even notice can either signal politeness or cause huge offence. Roles make a difference too: if one of my children complains to me about an ailment, I listen in a way that is entirely different to how I would listen to a patient. All listening, and all hearing, are innately selective.

In a professional context, I suspect that what we call good listening is in reality a process of conscious, decisive, and closely monitored tuning out. Good listeners may in fact be the people who are exceptionally aware of missing a great deal, accept that this is inevitable, and act accordingly. They manage to make deliberate choices, rather than accidental ones, about what to hear and not hear. They know that some words are clearly weighted by important markers such as repetition, intonation or emotion whereas other words are – relatively speaking – just noise. Conversely, bad listeners (apart from those who just can't be bothered) may be those who are possessed by the illusion that they can catch everything if they try hard enough. They treat all words as equal, and so they end up responding to random cues rather than significant ones.

Words, however, are not all. True listening involves many organs of sensation apart from the ears. Most obviously, people's faces and bodies speak to us just as much as their voices if not more. Most doctors will be aware of changes that can take place in the atmosphere of the consulting room, even in the smell. Many will be familiar with a range of alterations in their own physical state during consultations, ranging from a sense of calm to an urgent desire to pass wind. This too is information, in the form of what psychiatrists call counter-transference. During the moments in consultations when doctors are not actually listening in the literal sense, we are almost certainly picking up vast amounts of this kind of information, although we may be doing so at a purely intuitive level. We may even connect such impressions with something the patient has actually said, and later convince ourselves that we have acted only upon what we have 'heard'.

There is another process that is common in consultations too: the active decision to stop listening when we have heard as much as we need to know. Obviously this can be done crassly, and often is, especially when doctors lose interest in their patients as soon as they have established the diagnosis. But there is also a more creative way of withdrawing one's attention. It occurs when you need time to formulate something appropriate to say to the patient by way of medical information or advice, and you know that you will do better if you have an internal conversation with yourself rather than continuing to try and listen to what the patient is saying.

I had exactly this experience recently when a patient had told me enough for me to feel quite certain that the palpitations he was getting while at work arose from anxiety alone. Having reached this view, I knew that listening to any further narrative from him might make it harder for me to put this proposition to him, rather than easier. I ignored the rest of what he was saying, and used the time instead to choose a form of words in my own mind that I hoped he might find palatable and helpful. The stratagem seemed to work, and I found a way of putting my idea to him that he readily accepted, rather than insisting on lots of physical tests, as I feared he might. I don't think I would have achieved this if I had slavishly followed every detail of his lament. I might never have got onto his wavelength unless I had done exactly what my psychologist friend had done so expertly: tuning out.

32

END OF THE ROAD

....

We were not, at the time, living in our own house. We had a problem there with subsidence, so we had moved into an apartment elsewhere while the house was underpinned. However, on that particular Sunday afternoon we had come back to check how the work was progressing, and to pick up our mail. We found a parking place round the corner and then walked back to our home. As we did so, I registered in my mind – fleetingly, almost subliminally – that there was someone sitting on the pavement near the corner. A young black girl with a small suitcase. Walking on, I managed to adjust the image to something more precise: a forlorn child, sitting alone with her possessions, and possibly scared. After we had let ourselves into the house, I told my wife that I was concerned about the girl. My wife, six months pregnant and uncomfortable, had scarcely noticed her, but agreed to walk back up the street by herself and find out if anything was amiss. A few minutes later she returned to the house with the girl, and the suitcase.

It was clear that things were very much amiss. The girl, no more than thirteen years old, spoke no English and was almost too frightened to enter an empty and unfurnished house with two complete strangers. With gestures, we managed to indicate our good will and we brought her in. We also managed to deduce, from her looks and one or two words, that she was Ethiopian. One of the blessings of working in London general practice is that you become close to patients from many countries. I had several Ethiopian patients whom I knew well and could trust. I managed to find the phone number of one of these, a middle-aged woman with teenage children herself. I called her to ask if she could speak with the girl and find out what was going on. She willingly did so, and soon established how the girl had come to be sitting on our street corner.

The girl was apparently a domestic servant for a wealthy family from Saudi Arabia. They had brought her over with them on a holiday to London, but had then become displeased with her and abandoned her with a few belongings when they left their hotel. She had started to walk, in the hope that God might lead her to some kind of rescuer. When she reached our street – five or six miles from where she started – she had become exhausted and stopped to wait for whatever fate had in store. She knew nothing about the current whereabouts of any of her own family, who had all dispersed from eastern Ethiopia in different directions during the war there. She asked my patient for reassurance that my wife and I had good intentions, and were not scheming to force her into prostitution.

Over the phone, I discussed with my patient what we should do. She made the offer I had hoped she would: to take the girl in before registering her with the authorities the following day. We drove the girl over to their home, had tea with the family, thanked them for their kindness, and left her there. Over the next few days I stayed in contact with them as they notified social services and supported the girl as she was transferred into residential care. A couple of weeks later I received a rather chilling phone call from a social worker who grilled me about my own role in the matter: why had I not immediately called the police, how could I be certain that my own patient was not an abuser, was I aware of child protection procedures... and so forth. To be honest, absolutely none of these issues had even crossed my mind. I replied curtly that I had been acting as a citizen and not in a professional capacity. I restrained myself from telling her that I taught on child protection courses, or from asking where her own humanity lay.

In various ways I kept abreast of the girl's circumstances. She passed through a couple of foster homes, but stayed friends with the Ethiopian family who had been her first hosts. I saw her on a couple of further occasions, and she was clearly developing into a bright, feisty and alarmingly westernised teenager with an appropriately cool fashion sense. It is now nearly many since we found her. I imagine her to be probably a graduate, perhaps starting out on a professional career, possibly involved in political action on behalf of others. When I think back on twenty-five years of doing general practice, I can remember few more vivid or more positive moments than introducing her into the care of my patient that Sunday afternoon. And I remain mystified – as one always does – by the merciful influences that led her to sit down at the corner of our street at a particular moment on that Sunday afternoon.

33

ESCAPING THE
LOOP

....

This is a story about intuition and its relation to logic.

A mother came to see me with her nine-year-old son, who wets his bed. She wanted me to write a letter to the council to support the family's application for a bigger flat. The boy apparently has two elder brothers who share his bedroom. They are fed up with the smell of his urine and want another bedroom. When she made this request, I tensed up. I felt caught in a double bind. If I said no, I would probably lose any chance of helping the boy with his bedwetting. If I said yes, I would effectively be offering an incentive for his behaviour.

Like most doctors when faced with this kind of dilemma, I found a solution intuitively. But afterwards I analysed what I had done and realised that it conformed rather well with communication theory. This was a relief. I was in the middle of preparing a seminar on this topic for a group of doctors and beginning to have my doubts about whether it fitted real life. I will tell you about my solution later, but let me go into a little bit of the theory first.

When the philosophers Bertrand Russell and Alfred North Whitehead wrote a work called *Principia Mathematica* at the beginning of the last century, they proposed a Theory of Logical Types. A central argument of that theory was that a category 'cannot belong to itself'. To use the annoying language that philosophers love, the category of 'cats' is not a cat. More important, from the point of view of logic, the category of 'categories' is not itself a mere category. It is at a higher level of abstraction.

What this means in ordinary language is that categories of ideas or things have to nest inside each other like Russian dolls. They cannot ooze into each other like the protrusions of an amoeba, or suddenly leap to another level like excited electrons. At first sight this may seem obvious or seriously uninteresting, but it matters in philosophy because it helps people to identify and disprove certain errors of logic.

A generation after Russell and Whitehead, the theory was taken up by the biologist Gregory Bateson. He suggested that logical typing is a natural as well as a mathematical phenomenon. He argued that mammals, including humans, seem to display in their communications an intuitive understanding of logical levels. They particularly show evidence of this in the ways that they respond to the same stimuli in different ways according to different contexts.

One example is the mock fighting that occurs among young animals. Cubs of many species can bite each other in ways that look just like real fights, but because they give out signals of a 'higher level of context' that this is only play, no one gets hurt. If the signals about context get confused, no one knows which is the higher one, fighting or playing. The situation then gets frightening and nasty. You can see this logical confusion when children of a certain age are practising their aggression but then lose control.

Another example is humour. Bateson argued that humour is often the consequence of an intentional confusion of context levels. We recognise this as a logical trick even though we may not quite understand how it works, and we find it amusing. (For instance, I once looked at a Japanese print of an elephant and commented that I didn't think that there were elephants in Japan. 'But this isn't a real elephant,' the owner quipped. 'It's only a print of one!')

Bateson's ideas about logical typing in nature were taken up in their turn by communication theorists. They looked at conversations, and found that these tended to be harmonious if everyone shared the same assumptions about which context had the higher authority in any situation. However, things could become dysfunctional if this wasn't the case. For example, if one partner in a couple thinks that arguments are fine because there is an overarching commitment to work things out, while the other partner believes they define a relationship as a failing one, there will be trouble.

Returning now to my own difficult consultation, it is clear that there were two contexts vying for supremacy. One was 'the doctor as healer' and the other was 'the doctor as patient's advocate'. Whichever context I chose, I would automatically disqualify the other, and therefore fail in a legitimate part of my job. In communication theory, this is called a 'strange loop'.

Intuitively, I managed to get myself out of the loop. I said I was happy to write the letter but not yet. I wanted the boy first of all to attend the local enuresis clinic, and the family to make a serious attempt to engage with the treatment offered. If this failed, I would certainly back their application. The mother agreed at once. My guess is that the solution appealed to her in the context of 'the mother who wants a healthy child'. She was now able to set this above the alternative context of 'the mother who wants better accommodation' without having to let go of it altogether.

Of course the lure of better housing may lead the family in the end to sabotage any treatment, but I hope it will not. When there are strange loops around, disentangling them will often produce relief – and a feeling that intuition was the quickest route to discovering the logic. It often is.

34

IMPALED ON THE INVISIBLE

....

Driving into work, I was listening to the radio. Someone was talking about global warming, and quoting a statement from the Confederation of British Industry. 'Any measures taken to prevent global warming', went the statement, 'must not do any harm to British industry.' My ears pricked up. I wondered if anyone would challenge this, but of course no one did. Yet an intelligent ten-year-old could tell you that you cannot reduce global warming without harming industry. Conversely, if you do not take measures that will harm some industries, there will almost certainly be more global warming. That indeed is the dilemma.

Later the same day, I came across a similar argument. A friend asked me to look at an article he was writing about refugees and the restrictions being placed on their use of the NHS in Britain. I read the article. It was passionate and polemical, but I doubted if it would convince anyone who was not already convinced. I asked my friend provocatively if he was proposing to open Britain and its health service to anyone in the world, regardless of their nationality or level of need. (He looked troubled for a moment. I don't normally ask such illiberal questions.) I pointed out that his article was similar to the statement I had heard on the radio. It involved the denial of a dilemma.

Denied dilemmas are incredibly common. Once you start noticing them, you spot them everywhere. Politics is almost entirely based on them. Every speech, every manifesto, is either for something or against it. Certainly, very few politicians – at least in public – seem able to frame any issue as a painful dilemma and to confess that they are proposing what they hope, on the balance of probabilities, to be the 'least worst' option. (*'My fellow Americans, we are going to fight a war. Perhaps it will lead to peace in the Middle East, and perhaps it will make things worse. We may be saving more lives, or putting more at risk. I simply ask you to back my hunch that on balance this is the right thing to do …'*)

In theory at least, doctors are in a very different position from politicians. We are not obliged by our calling to take up postures where we deny the existence of dilemmas. Nor do we have to conceal any private doubts we may have, in order to stay in our jobs. In spite of this, I believe that we may not be any better at spotting dilemmas, or naming them, than politicians are.

One particularly fashionable way for doctors to deny dilemmas these days is for them to quote scientific evidence in a way that implies that it abolishes any possibility of a dilemma (*'Studies show that these pills will lower your chances of a heart attack'*). In fact, this tactic is usually lazy, ignorant or disingenuous. The more we acquire evidence, the more we should actually become aware of alternative options, and therefore of the need to offer complex choices to patients. (*'If you do "x", these are the likely consequences. If you do "y", these are the different consequences. Or you could do nothing and this is what might follow.'*) Contrary to what many doctors seem to believe, evidence-based medicine should lead us away from certainty and closer to decisions that are based on patients' preferences, values and intuition.

I spend a fair amount of time offering supervision to other doctors, and as I listen to the anxious stories that they bring about cases that are upsetting them, I find denied dilemmas popping up all over the place. Often, the doctors who present cases have understood their problems in terms of conflict, but not as dilemmas. Asking people to reframe their problems as dilemmas can have a quite instant effect, sometimes with a visible jolt, as clarity replaces muddle. ('*If I declare this patient unfit for work I'm not being honest. But if I refuse, I may lose his co-operation.*') Often, such a reframing will lead to a resolution to hand the dilemma back fairly and squarely to where it belongs: with the patient.

From observation of doctors who appear in the mass media, it seems that members of our profession find it hard to admit that every medical issue has its dilemmas, however obvious the facts or the science may seem. The most solid of medical truths are only provisional, and ultimately we can never free ourselves from the dilemma posed by our lack of foreknowledge: '*This is what we doctors believe at the moment, but we have made asses of ourselves in the past. To be honest, we may be making asses of ourselves again ...*'

35

WEASEL WORDS

....

Here is a conference advertisement that appeared recently:

> 'Choice Partnership presents Managing Care Services Improvement: a two day conference exploring citizenship, new realities, and sharing risk through promoting integrated delivery of health, housing and social services.'

Fascinated by the language, I decided I would put some of the phrases on cards, shuffle them, ask my wife to pick up cards at random, and then put the resulting sequence of phrases back into the original framework. We did the exercise three times. This is what we came up with:

A. 'New Realities Partnership presents Managing Choice: a two day conference exploring care services improvement, health, housing and social care services, and promoting sharing risk through integrated delivery of citizenship.'

B. 'Care Services Improvement Partnership presents Managing New Realities: a two day conference exploring choice, sharing risk and promoting citizenship through integrated delivery of health, housing and social care services.'

C. 'Sharing Risk Partnership presents Managing Health, Housing and Social Care Services: a two day conference exploring new realities, care services improvement, and promoting choice through integrated delivery of citizenship.'

Now I have to confess I have played a little trick on you. The original advertisement was actually not the one in the first paragraph but version B... or possibly C, or maybe A. Can you guess which one? Of course not. Because the genuine version is just as vacuous as the scrambled ones. They are all equally devoid of meaning, a kind of political pornography, designed to induce a satisfied glow of righteous recognition in the same way that a photo of two breasts or a bottom is calculated to produce a different kind of glow.

Why do we not scream with outrage at the constant assault we now suffer from this kind of language in the public services? Or even better, why do we not laugh at it till the tears stream down our cheeks? It reminds me of spending a morning not too long ago in the presence of a score of senior colleagues while we all struggled with the question set for us by a highly paid facilitator: how were we going to rise to the challenge of consumer choice, a patient-led service, an accelerated pace of change coupled with necessary efficiency savings? We all sat there like well-behaved children at an old-fashioned preparatory school, listening to this rubbish as if it meant anything. By the end of the morning we were actually *speaking* the stuff, as if we believed it, as if it had become part of us. Grown men and women, each with decades of serious professional experience, were jumping up energetically to add empty resolutions to the bullet points on two flip charts, under the fatuous headings of 'quick wins' and 'smart objectives'. For goodness' sake, what is happening to us? Can anything be done to prevent us losing our souls entirely to this fraudulent drivel?

Before I decline into permanent acquiescence with it, let me spell out some truths that may help us resist this pervasive deceit in the public services:

1. There is a close relationship between corruption of language, corruption of thought, and corruption of action. There may be some ways in which parts of the public services are improving at any given time, and it is even possible that some organisational changes may be for the better. However, celebrating these patchy successes in increasingly messianic slogans leads to the disablement of any serious analysis, then to the denial of any error or failure, and then to systematic cover-up and abuse.

2. It used not to be like this. There was a time in the recent past when people in the West read such bombast with horror, because we thought it belonged to totalitarian states where people were unable to protest at the blatant hypocrisy that surrounded them.

3. The practice of medicine is not a state activity, and doctors who are over-identified with the state, or with the language of the state, have sold out. Medicine is generally conservative and respectful of those in power, and it probably needs to be. But there are also times when medicine has to be subversive. Doctors who cannot act, think and speak subversively can be dangerous.

4. Thank goodness, we still live in a society where we can at least make fun of people in positions of power who tell lies to themselves or others, who take themselves too seriously, or who talk nonsense. We should take every opportunity to do so. As most of the population of Europe discovered during the twentieth century, it is a right that is quickly and easily removed, and only recovered at an appalling cost.

36

FOLK ILLNESS AND MEDICAL MODELS

....

Sometimes an author manages to capture the essence of an article with such an arresting name that you feel compelled to read it. A few years ago I was scanning a list of references when I came across a title so striking that I went to a library at once, to read through the article in question and see if it lived up to its promise. It was called 'Hyper-Tension: a folk illness with a medical name'. The author of the paper was the American social anthropologist Dan Blumhagen. I was not disappointed. I now regard it as one of the most enlightening pieces of social science research that I have ever read. And although it is nearly forty years old – an aeon in terms of most academic writing – I still use it when teaching doctors and asking them to think about their patients' medical ideas and their own.

Blumhagen reported on how he interviewed 117 men attending a hypertension clinic over a period of twelve months, in order to establish their beliefs about the condition. While all the doctors were clear that hypertension was simply another word for high blood pressure, he found that patients – while knowing the two were somehow connected – all had an idea in their minds that it meant something far more complex. Blumhagen gave this idea the name of

'Hyper-Tension'. He found that each person appeared to have an individual model of what had caused their Hyper-Tension, together with a collection of ideas about how their body had reacted, and a further set of ideas about symptoms and risks. For example, in one typical individual the causes of hypertension included 'family arguments', the physical reaction was described as 'ballooning veins', the symptoms were felt as 'dizzy spells and flashing lights', and the patient feared the possibility of a ruptured blood vessel, leading to 'loss of a kidney'.

Blumhagen found that many of these individual models seemed to have a great deal in common, so that he was able to draw up a visual map of the 'folk illness', linking together fifty-seven concepts such as 'acute stress', 'narrowed blood vessels', 'heart attack' and so forth, with arrows of various thickness indicating the direction of causation as understood by a significant number of people.

No doctor who treats hypertension will be surprised by these findings, particularly the strong belief that the patients seemed to have in the psychological origins of high blood pressure, and the almost universal (if incorrect) belief that hypertension usually causes symptoms. But the real fascination of Blumhagen's work is in the discussion that surrounds these findings. It is impossible to do full justice to this here, not least because the article is thirty pages long, but a few indications of the argument may give an impression of its richness.

First, Blumhagen challenges the idea that 'folk' beliefs are entirely separate from 'formal' medical ones. He proposes instead that the two are closely interdependent, the popular condition of 'Hyper-Tension' clearly echoing the expert one, while at the same drawing on associations with more familiar words such as 'tension' and 'pressure'. He also demonstrates how any individual's beliefs are often inconsistent or may change rapidly. For instance, someone might describe 'stress' as a cause of their hypertension, yet later in the same conversation, when focussing on a different aspect of their experience, describe it as a consequence. Or alternatively, as Blumhagen says, 'if one inquires about the physical causes of an illness, an explanatory model may be given which will be radically different from the explanatory model given by the same individual if one then asks about the spiritual or social causes of the same illness'.

In other words, what patients bring us when they talk about their illnesses is not some rigid and fully considered theory, but rather a loosely connected and fluctuating bundle of ideas, apprehensions and word associations, often oriented towards justifying a particular aspect of behaviour (for example, taking pills or not taking them, working hard or taking early retirement, and so on).

All of this certainly helps to make sense of what goes on in everyday consultations, not just with high blood pressure but with many other conditions. However, the main challenge that Blumhagen presents is to propose that the official medical model of 'real' hypertension may bear a great deal of resemblance to the folk version. He shows, for example, how the published medical literature presents a constant reworking of our professional models and belief systems, so that obsolete ideas slide imperceptibly out of view as if they had never been there, while new ones are written into the story in their place – each successive version being presented, of course, as an ultimate truth.

Similarly, he demonstrates how different practitioners present their patients with versions of the 'facts' about high blood pressure that are highly personal and selective in terms of what they include, omit or emphasise. Such explanations, although delivered with great professional conviction, mainly seem to serve the purpose of supporting the advice or treatment the doctor has already decided to give. These explanations also contain the same inconsistencies that you find with patients: for instance, a doctor might at one moment reassure someone that high blood pressure is unrelated to a stressful life style, while in the next breath offering the standard inane advice to 'try to relax more' or to 'avoid stress'.

Social scientists often tend to write about medicine in a way that can leave the ordinary jobbing doctor with a sense of futility and a wish to phone the pensions agency for an estimate at the first opportunity, but surprisingly Blumhagen ends on a more positive note:

'Plain folk say "Hyper-Tension"; the experts say hypertension, and each thinks the other is talking about the same thing. Perhaps it is this muddying of the waters which allows both to function without cognitive dissonance becoming so great as to cut off interaction... But there are occasions when dissonance caused by different models of illness does impede healing. At those times, a full understanding of the illness belief systems which are available to the layman and to the physician, if coupled with a willingness to negotiate a more functional set of explanatory models, may pave the way to a richer, deeper and above all more satisfying experience to healing.'

37

THE FACTS OF
DEATH

....

I have lost two friends to pancreatic cancer recently. Two other friends are in the middle of cancer treatment and unsure what the outcome will be for them. From all these friends, and from many others who have had cancer in the past, I have heard the same stories. Their medical care has been excellent in technical terms, but personally it has been stony cold. However often we remark on the fact, it still remains true that doctors are mostly not good about death and dying. Although death is the sole certainty for every patient that we see, and very few people in Western society will die without a doctor in attendance during their final days, we still treat the whole business of death as if it is an aberration, a failure, or something that doesn't really belong to medicine at all.

In cancer clinics and on the wards, the prevailing way of speaking with patients who have fatal illnesses appears to be efficient at best, and defensive or avoidant at worst. Different members of the medical teams come and go, often without any introduction or explanation of their role in the system. Each doctor delivers a partial message – a test result, or a new treatment option – but no one appears to hold the whole case together. Nobody, least of all the senior consultants, ever seems to sit down and take time to speak the truths that really matter: 'Our treatment may delay your death but it cannot prevent it', 'I'm sorry but our treatment hasn't worked'. It doesn't matter whether patients are attending local hospitals or major teaching centres, or even whether they are doctors themselves. Only when people reach a hospice – if they are lucky enough to do so – does it seem as if most professionals start to shed their embarrassment, annoyance or fear, and start to behave like human beings.

Hospices, of course, place death and dying at the centre of their work, but I wonder what would happen if we did this for all of medicine. It would certainly make sense to see everything that we do as doctors in terms of managing mortality, or as deferring death rather than defeating it. Since no one lives for ever, all medical interventions are really just attempts to buy time, or to make time pass more comfortably.

We could in fact think of our work as falling essentially into three categories. There is preventative treatment, which may lower people's statistical risk of a disease, but will make no difference to the vast majority of people being treated, who would never have acquired the disease anyway. Then there are routine treatments like antibiotics, which are used far more often than they need to be, generally for conditions that would have improved by themselves. Finally, there are a few treatments that can be genuinely life-saving, but still cannot prolong life indefinitely. Even this last category of treatment (for example, cardiac surgery) is increasingly used for elderly people, prolonging their lives only for a relatively short time.

If we put death at the centre of medicine, we would also need to give the facts of death a proper place in medical training. We would then learn that, in evolutionary terms, death is just as much part of our existence as sex. There is in fact an increasing amount of evidence that the two are entirely interdependent. Primitive creatures such as bacteria, which evolved before sex appeared on the world scene, multiply without sex. However, they also do not die automatically in the way we do. Instead, they only perish when the environment around them changes, for example when water or salt disappears, or when the temperature changes. When sexual reproduction arrived, about a billion years after the bacteria, pre-determined death arrived alongside it. In other words, at the same time that genes gained the ability to merge with each other through sexual conjunction, they also evolved the ability to kill the creatures they made. We commonly call genes 'selfish', but this doesn't just mean that they will find every possible means to promote their own replication. It also means that in time they will destroy each of us as individuals, once we have fulfilled our task of reproducing them – or at least been given the opportunity to do so.

The question as to why older people die should, we now know, be turned on its head if we want a satisfactory answer. The real explanation lies in the corollary: young people, generally speaking, almost never die from natural causes. While we are young, the more deadly genes that we all carry, and that will inevitably see us off one day, are counteracted by protective genes that keep them at bay until we have had a chance to do our reproductive duty. If the protective genes were less effective they would let us perish before we could reproduce, and hence would have become extinct. Equally, if the same protective genes were more effective and operated over a longer period of the life cycle, they would have left the world cluttered up with elderly individuals past their reproductive potential, but consuming resources that could be better used for younger individuals who are still fertile. The death genes and the protective genes keep the balance between sex and death permanently at just the right level.

As far as cancer is concerned, it seems a fair guess that each of us is born with genes that can induce some of our cells to run out of control and proliferate, in the form of malignant tumours. What holds this at bay in most of us probably has little to do with our physical lifestyle, let alone our moral attitude, and far more to do with the needs of our sex cells: the sperm and eggs that combine to create the next generation. These sex cells differ in many respects from all our other cells (the so-called somatic cells). One of these differences is that sex cells are much better at repairing their own DNA when it become damaged. By the time we are old, a very small selection of our extra-resilient sperm or eggs will therefore usually have departed elsewhere to perpetuate some of our genes in the form of our children, but will have left behind a large number of less robust somatic cells with the capacity to multiply and kill us, or at least to degenerate to the point where they are no longer viable.

This is a sombre view of life. In a book entitled *Sex and the Origins of Death*, the immunologist William Clark sums it up as follows: 'We want so desperately to be more than just a vehicle for DNA, and at least transiently we are. Yet somatic cells will die at the end of each generation, whether they are part of an insect wing or a human brain. We may come to understand death, but we cannot change this single, simple fact: in the larger scheme of things, it matters not a whit that some of these somatic cells contain all that we hold most dear about ourselves; our ability to think, to feel, to love – to write and read these very words. In terms of the basic process of life itself, which is the transmission of DNA from one generation to the next, all of this is so much sound and fury, signifying certainly very little, and quite possibly nothing.'

There is a danger that such a view might lead many doctors to take an even more indifferent and unfeeling approach to their dying patients than they already do. Yet perhaps if it were taught more widely, the same view could also form the basis of greater compassion, and a greater sense of participation in the face of the one fate we all share. Some of the best doctors I know have always questioned much that passes for medical treatment. They have had no illusions about the temptation we face every day, to imply – through omission, distortion, or downright lies – that we can avert the inevitable. A better knowledge of the nature and purpose of death might help more doctors to see medicine in its rightful perspective, and to talk straightforwardly and compassionately to their patients about what we can and cannot do. It is medicine that is peripheral to death, not the other way around.

38

CARE PATHWAYS

....

If you want to use the main car park and can afford to pay up to £25 a day to do so, you may be lucky enough to spot the sign to the main entrance of Bleakston General Hospital. If you come by public transport, however, you will have to ask the bus driver where to get off because the nearest stop is about ten minutes' walk away, by the hospital's back entrance. Even when you are off the bus, you can struggle to find it because it is barely signposted. Your best bet is to follow other people, mainly elderly, as they wait patiently by the pedestrian crossing for the lights to change and then stumble their way across as hastily as they are able.

Reaching the back entrance, there is a large sign saying 'Accident and Emergency Only: No Access to Main Hospital'. Fortunately you will sometimes find a security guard there who will point you towards a small unmarked door that leads to a connecting corridor. Inside the corridor, there is at least a helpful arrow saying 'All Departments'. As you walk down the corridor, you notice various assorted signs. For example, there is a yellow plastic sign saying 'Neuro-radiology', an ancient painted one saying 'Theatre staff only', and a piece of A4 paper stuck on with sticky putty saying 'HR department turn left'. There are also doors and staircases with no notices at all. Nowhere is there a map.

Eventually you come across a sign to 'Oncology Reception'. Although that is not your destination, you hope you might find someone helpful at the desk. Alas, the young woman is clearly annoyed at being used all the time as a general information bureau. She responds to your request for directions by inquiring sarcastically why you didn't come in at the main entrance and ask there. Grudgingly, she tells you that you can reach your destination by going down the stairs behind you and following signs to 'Block B'.

The stairs take you down to a corridor with heating pipes along it. There are stray items abandoned along it, including hospital trolleys and antique wheelchairs. At the end of the corridor is another set of stairs, leading up to a large yard. One side of the yard consists of the original Victorian workhouse that still contains some of the old wards. On the other side of the yard is a ramp leading to a 1980s tower block. The concrete is stained and pitted and the block already looks more dilapidated than its nineteenth-century neighbour. Elsewhere around the yard you can see several portakabins, a building site with a crane and piles of rubble. But there are no further signs showing where you might find Block B...

Every week I visit at least one hospital in the course of my work. On almost every occasion I have an experience similar to the one above. The description I have given has been combined from several recent visits, and represents the average. Sometimes things are slightly better and sometimes they are worse, but I am usually relieved to have given myself an extra half hour to find the venue for my meeting. It is surprising how often there is no public transport taking you direct to the main entrance. The lack of thoughtful and consistent signposting is almost universal, even in newly built hospitals. So is architectural disorder ranging from inconsistency to absolute chaos. Sadly, it is also a regular experience to meet reception staff who are abrupt or rude when asked for information outside their paid remit.

One thing that strikes me about these experiences is the lack of imagination they represent on the part of some hospital managers. If a visitor like myself – healthy, alert, unrushed, and on official business – finds myself disoriented and upset, what on earth must it be like for someone older, frail, anxious, unwell, and late for an appointment? Alongside a failure of imagination, I suspect there is a failure of responsibility too. I wonder how many hospitals could identify a single person who is in charge of making the overall experience of the visitor a tolerable one. Surely someone could wander around any hospital now and again with an observant eye – or even accompanied by an outsider – to make sure that everything is easy to find, and that topographical muddles are made intelligible through maps, colour codes or other aids.

Thoughtful managers could no doubt make a lot of difference, but the problem goes deeper than management. Almost everything I have described is a symbol – and often a direct outcome – of the way we approach health and the health service in Britain. The inadequacy of public transport and the scandalous costs of hospital parking are not an accident or a coincidence. They are the results of calculated policy decisions, and a national state of indifference to inequality. The bewildering layout of hospitals simply compounds the difficulty of getting an appointment in the first place, because of waiting lists and scarce resources. The confusion and incoherence of hospital architecture stand as metaphors for inconsistent health policies, sudden shifts of political direction and a lack of long-term strategic planning. The rudeness of reception staff, albeit inexcusable, is a token of demoralisation and deprofessionalisation in the public services. Somehow the notion of providing a friendly, caring service to the public has lost out to the idea that patients should be grateful for what they get.

But perhaps the explanation for these experiences lies deeper still. It often strikes me how hospitals can resemble the diseases they are offering to treat. The peeling walls or disintegrating concrete call to mind eczema or psoriasis. The proliferation of different styles of building, spread around at random, seems like a form of uncontrolled cancer. The most disorienting hospital I have come across was one of London's last remaining mental hospitals, laid out in locked and unmarked buildings over an enormous acreage of land: it took the best part of an hour to locate anyone there who was expecting me, and who knew why I had come or where I should be going. A patient who was not already feeling depersonalised, fragmented and excluded on arrival there would surely feel that way within a very short time.

It must be an illusion to think that we can make people's bodies and minds better irrespective of the environment in which we try to do so. Patients whose moods are affected by the thoughtlessness, ugliness and impoverishment of their surroundings cannot be in a state of mind to join as partners in their treatment. If we want to convince people that we can make them better, we should be able to give them signs – in every sense – that we know where they are coming from, and where they should be going. If we mean to make the patient's journey as painless as possible, we need to start, quite literally, at the bus stop.

39

ON KINDNESS

....

'I'm not a clever doctor, but I am a kind one.' My colleague's statement was striking and I have remembered it for many years. He was another local GP, close to retirement, and I was interviewing him as part of a research project. Everything I had learned about him during the conversation supported what he said. He wasn't a high earner by comparison with most GPs, mainly because he cared little for ticking the boxes on lucrative but clinically pointless targets set by the government or local managers. However, his consulting room walls were covered with framed photos of weddings and new babies from among the families he cared for, and his window sill was hidden underneath dozens of thank you cards. I discovered that he was now looking forward to retirement because it would allow him to be a full-time grandparent to his daughter's little boy and girl whom he adored – but at the same time he was worried that his former patients might fall into the hands of a younger GP of the sort who might install a large, visible clock in the consulting room, or who might think it improper to take someone's hand in sympathy.

When the interview had finished he escorted me out through the waiting room. His evening session was about to start. He greeted each of the patients with a friendly smile or a touch on the shoulder. I sensed no element of sentimentality or theatre in this. It was the quality he had himself identified as his main strength: kindness. I wondered how many more doctors like him I would ever meet before the numbing effects of bureaucracy and defensive medicine became universal and made this way of practising unknown. I also wondered how many of us would ever look back on our careers as doctors and make a similar judgement of ourselves. In my own case, I could certainly remember significant acts of kindness that I felt proud of, but I could also recall an equal number of occasions – if not more – when I performed my tasks in a spirit of irritable efficiency, doing what was right because I knew this intellectually rather than through genuine warmth. Perhaps this barely mattered for much of the time: the prescription I wrote might have achieved the same result anyway. But I have no doubt that there were many occasions when the missing ingredient was the crucial one, and patients failed to engage with my advice or to follow it through because it seemed disengaged and mechanical – or because they believed that soulless medicine couldn't be trusted.

An article in the *British Medical Journal* makes this point even more forcefully. In a piece entitled 'The kindness of strangers', the medical director of a hospice describes the death of her father, and then of her life partner and soulmate. She tells of how 'an invisible, untaught web of kindness and generosity' was spun around each of these losses. In the rest of the article she offers her thoughts on the new national end of life strategy in England, and on measurable outcomes. She laments our over-reliance on online learning and competency tests, arguing that these are no substitute for wise decision-making and kindness. She reflects on what outcomes might be truly meaningful. 'I could think of only two', she writes. '"Did I hear what matters most for this person right now?" and "Was I kind?"'

As an educator, I was arrested by this article too. We pay a lot of attention to language and emotion, but I cannot remember ever using the words 'wisdom' and 'kindness' in a seminar or lecture. Since reading the article, I have started to imagine what it would be like if we made these virtues transparent in our teaching rather than implicit, or if we were bold enough to point out that the best communication techniques in the world are empty without them. I have also been thinking about whether we should assess kindness as an important outcome of medical training. As well as observing whether students followed verbal feedback and body language, perhaps we could also ask 'were they kind?'

I am sure there would be risks in doing so. It might reward those with advanced skills as actors, rather than those with genuine compassion. Kindness could also wither under observation, through some kind of Heisenberg principle of the emotions. Yet we could certainly inquire about it after real professional encounters, where it would be harder to fake it. When seeking opinions from patients for appraisal purposes, as we often do nowadays, it might be possible to include the simple question, 'How far were you treated with wisdom, and with kindness?'

Kindness in individuals is important, but spreading kindness across whole organisations may be even more so. In this regard, there are useful lessons to be learned from an initiative that took place in Indiana University a few years ago, when a team of researchers and volunteers undertook the exercise of changing patterns of interaction across an entire medical school. Although they did not set out to produce kindness, this is exactly what they achieved.

The researchers began by holding interviews with a large selection of students, residents, fellows, faculty and staff. They asked these people to identify narratives of positive experiences from their working lives, and recorded these systematically. By doing this, they hoped to capture peak moments at work, rather than dwelling on critical incidents and negative perceptions. The most striking effect of the research was how much it brought out feelings of closeness, respect, joy and hope for interviewee and interviewer alike. When the team presented the narratives in public, the medical school community was reminded of 'its deep reservoirs of caring about patients and students'.

One participant is quoted as saying afterwards: 'Now that I see how good we really are, I have to ask myself why we tolerate it when people aren't as good as this. I can't look on quietly any more when people are disrespectful or hurtful. It's no longer okay to remain silent; this is too important.' Another interesting finding was the linkage between the level of emotional care and the outcome of care in the technical sense. One faculty member, for example, described how he was able to manage a complex surgical case because of the amount of trust and honesty that were present among the clinicians, and with the patient and his family.

Following the initiative, there seemed to be a ripple effect in the medical school, with small acts of care and kindness spreading across the institution. At a subsequent committee meeting one participant simply rearranged the furniture to enable people to sit closer together. Another person was moved at a finance meeting to give voice to feelings of heartbreak at budget cuts, even though there was no precedent for such personal comments. A senior faculty member was observed making a significant detour from his path to the hospital parking garage to escort a 'lost-looking couple' to their destination. Complimentary remarks and emails became commoner across the whole medical school.

The authors analyse these consequences in terms of a theory known as Complex Responsive Processes. According to this theory, small changes in behaviour can sometimes spread quickly and widely, transforming patterns of thinking and interaction across an organisation. The theory encourages those who want to change their workplaces to focus not on 'elaborate idealised designs' but instead to participate positively in here-and-now interactional processes.

I find the research impressive, and the theory is persuasive. It also makes sense simply at a human and intuitive level. I doubt if the GP whom I interviewed all those years ago would have needed any research, or any knowledge of theory, to behave as he did, or to realise it would make a difference to his patients and to their health. Perhaps being clever and being kind are not so different after all.

40

CAPABLE BUT
INSANE

....

For anyone who is interested in personal narratives of illness, it is hard to find one that is more remarkable than *Memoirs of My Nervous Illness* by Daniel Paul Schreber. Schreber was a judge in Germany at the end of the nineteenth century. He suffered from what we would now call paranoid schizophrenia. At the age of fifty-one he was admitted to a psychiatric asylum – first voluntarily, then under a court order – for nine years. Towards the end of this period he believed himself to be recovering, but his doctors did not take the same view. Although his behaviour was acceptable at this stage, it was clear to them that his ideas were still bizarre. He thus began a prolonged legal battle for his release. To support his case, he wrote a book-length account of his experiences and beliefs, which he subsequently expanded and then published. In the last few years this has been re-issued with an introduction by the writer Rosemary Dinnage, together with the medical reports that his psychiatrist submitted to the court and the final judgement releasing him to the outside world. It makes fascinating reading, not just for psychiatrists but for any doctor who may deal with disturbed people at times.

The opening pages set the tone for the book. They are articulate, compelling, coherent – and patently mad. Even though he felt he had recovered, Schreber still believed he had come under the influence of rays from the director of his previous asylum, Professor Flechsig. These rays were in turn a manifestation of rays from God, intended not only to make him suffer but to redeem the world and restore it to a state of Blessedness. As part of this redemptive process, he sometimes experienced his penis turning inwards in order to transform into a womb and ovaries, with the aim of allowing him to repopulate the world. Within what Dinnage describes as 'the complicated, mythic universe that Schreber in his captivity created', there are not only rays and miracles, but upper and lower gods, souls and soul murder, voices of nerve language, and struggles against the 'Order of the World'. There are speculations on the nature of God and of the different religions. Schreber describes how his mind was possessed or populated at various times by Benedictine monks, Jesuits, the Eternal Jew and a Mongolian prince.

Schreber gives some very precise and persuasive accounts of common mental phenomena, including aural hallucinations and intrusive thoughts. For example, at one point he describes how external voices may repeat certain phrases to him over and over again, but with the same word missing each time so that he feels compelled to complete the phrase by saying it to himself. As Dinnage points out, we are given insights into the development and nature of a healthy mind, through being granted such a detailed and privileged description of one that has become 'forsaken', to use Schreber's own word. There is some guidance, too, about what may help when people are in such desperate states of mind. This includes music, which at times seemed to Schreber to provide an alternative form of order, logic and language that was able to suppress the cacophony that generally persecuted him.

Schreber takes over two hundred and fifty pages to explain his entire delusional system – as we would regard it – although he makes it clear he can barely begin to give an account of his revelations in so short a space. Ultimately, he claims, these cannot really be expressed in words but are only available to intuition. His *Memoirs* certainly offer food for thought philosophically. He addresses some of the key questions that have taxed thinkers across the ages, including the nature of reality and how we know what truly exists. He does so in a manner that is clearly learned, with copious references including literary and scientific ones. There are moments when his manner of thinking appears to recall the kind of fringe religious cults that have always existed across the ages, and may even seem privy to hidden truths about the world. It isn't hard to imagine reading about his beliefs with curiosity rather than diagnosis in mind if, for example, they were reported as part of an anthropological account of a remote tribe.

The *Memoirs* have been subjected to many commentaries and judgements since they were first published. The most notable of these was from Freud, who believed that Schreber's disturbance arose from repressed homosexuality. Later, the liberal psychiatrist Thomas Szasz drew attention to how Schreber's incarceration and treatment may itself have amplified his disturbance. More recently, the focus of speculation has often been on Schreber's family and particularly on his father, Moritz, a noted authority of his time on child-rearing. Among the published guidance given by Schreber senior was the advice that children should have icy baths daily from the age of three months, be taught to obey their parents unquestioningly in all circumstances, and be strapped to special boards (marketed as the Schreber *Geradehalte*) if they slouched. His system was widely influential in Germany, and arguably contributed to the mindset that later made Nazism possible.

All of these hypotheses are interesting, although personally I find little direct evidence for any of them in the text or court reports. What I find more notable is the scrupulous attitude of Schreber's own psychiatrist, Dr Guido Weber, in the three submissions he wrote to the courts. In a careful, literate style, Weber emphasised more than once that his role was to describe and not to judge. He analysed the nature of Schreber's disordered thoughts but at the same time pointed out that such highly organised delusions could co-exist with normal social function. He even drew the sympathetic analogy of a gifted scientist who might hold passionate religious beliefs without them interfering with his scientific work, and with his colleagues entirely unaware of them. Even though he seems to have been opposed to Schreber's release, it is likely that Weber's even-handedness played a major part in leading the court to their surprisingly enlightened decision on appeal: 'The Court is in no doubt that the appellant is insane... [However] the Court of Appeal has arrived at the conviction that the plaintiff is capable of dealing with the demands of life in all its spheres.'

Schreber was a free man again, but his story does not have a happy ending. When his wife Sabine suffered a stroke, he had another breakdown, returned to the asylum, and stayed there until his death at the age of sixty-nine. Yet his *Memoirs* remain a model among illness narratives, and an example of just how much personal accounts can help us deepen our understanding of what patients experience.

41

ON THE RECORD

....

Doctors are prolific writers, often without realising it. We each spend a great deal of time writing in patient files or on computer records. During a medical career every one of us probably writes the equivalent of many full-length novels or even an encyclopaedia. We write automatically, often at great speed, drawing mainly on a repertoire of verbal formulas that we have learned from others, and imagining that all we are doing is writing down an objective record of what has happened. Yet our notes reveal more than we are aware of – not just about our patients but about ourselves and the wider culture in which we live. Medical notes written a century ago, carefully entered with pen and ink into leather-bound ward ledgers, are vastly different from the notes in modern case folders, bulging with computer printouts and copies of correspondence – let alone from the electronic medical records that are now taking over from these. The differences are testimony not only to changing technologies and scientific knowledge. They show radically altered forms of thinking and social relations as well.

A number of scholars in the last few years have looked closely at medical notes, examining how we listen selectively to patients' stories and transmute these into oral and written texts, often radically altering their meaning as we do so. One of the most impressive of these scholars is Petter Aaslestad, a professor of literature at Trondheim in Norway. During the 1990s he decided to apply his expertise as a literary critic to patient files. He took as his material a sample of a hundred sets of notes from 1890 onwards at Gaustad Hospital, the leading psychiatric hospital in Norway. His analysis was published in 1997 and soon become recognised in Scandinavia as a masterpiece. It is especially fascinating for anyone with an interest in the history of psychiatry. However, its originality and depth of thought make it relevant for anyone who ever writes notes about patients, or indeed anyone who has been a patient.

Aaslestad points out, for example, how doctors virtually never report patients' histories in their own uninterrupted words, or in direct quotations using the word 'I'. Instead, they diminish patients through a variety of distancing techniques, including a kind of telegrammatic writing that uses indirect speech and omits pronouns (e.g. 'feels unwell' instead of 'Mr N said, "I feel unwell."'). Similarly, although doctors always elicit case histories by systematic questioning, they rarely record the questions themselves. As a result, the notes generally create a false impression of giving a spontaneous patient narrative while actually following a logic dictated by the doctor.

Aaslestad also shows how doctors routinely characterise their patients by static and simplistic judgements ('calm and agreeable', 'utterly confused', 'extremely rude and challenging') rather than precise descriptions. He analyses how issues of gender, social class and power are embedded in the language of medical notes. Thus women are 'unhappy in love' while a man has 'an affair that went awry'. Similarly, lower-class patients are 'prone to drink', wealthier ones never so. If a patient has an influential relative, such as a member of parliament, this is dutifully recorded.

These textual details are only the starting point for some wider cultural observations. Aaslestad illustrates how medical notes sometimes echo the literary genres of their era, including the modernist novel and the detective story. Inevitably, they also reflect the beliefs and ideologies of their time. In one era religious belief is taken as a sign of virtue, whereas at a later time it is seen as cranky and suspect. The jargon of fashionable psychological theories, often in debased forms, seeps into and out of the texts, as doctors offer different and sometimes outrageous formulations of why patients behave as they do.

Many entries in the notes seem composed mainly in order to justify the diagnosis or treatment. If these change, the flow of the text is adjusted accordingly, so that the shifting medical narrative always provides the grounds for whatever the doctors are thinking or doing. In more recent years, individual entries seem to be addressed to a increasing variety of imagined readers including other doctors, the hospital authorities, or inspectorates. In a striking – and depressingly familiar – extract from modern times, the notes of one patient propose an extended stay at the time of his admission, but support his discharge shortly afterwards when there is a lack of space on the ward.

While there is some historical evolution of ideas and rhetorical positions over the course of the century examined by Aaslestad, certain features remain constant. One of these is the doctors' expressions of irritation when patients do not follow their treatment. Another is their incomprehension when patients take a different view of the world from their own. However, Aaslestad is also careful to explain the professional and cultural contexts that have influenced the entries in the notes. He makes a distinction between good and bad writers, and points out how 'a writer's warmth, ignorance, lack of manners, empathy, self-righteousness, humour or self-criticism, all leave traces, almost independently of the record's medical content'.

Perhaps the most telling example in the book is one from recent years. Here, a doctor describes a patient who has asked to see his own file, following a change in the law on freedom of information:

'He has seen it, and as he read it through he smiled several times and said, "I shan't comment on what it says, but I understand why you see it this way." It was impossible to get him to be specific about what he was reacting to.'

This patient's dignified silence, and his sense of the *impossibility* of getting professionals to understand his perspective in the way he understands theirs, speaks volumes. The extract offers support to a number of writers who now argue that patients shouldn't only have the right to read their own notes – something that few of them seem to have done, and with little effect. They should be able to write in them too.

Aaslestad argues convincingly that doctors need to become more aware of the political and cultural influences that govern their descriptions of patients, and to understand how oppressive these descriptions can become. In the words of one reviewer: 'This is a book for those of us who write patient files. Read it and consider how you describe your fellow beings.'

42

CLOSE READINGS

....

When I was at school I had an English teacher who taught us how to read literature very closely. We might spend a whole hour looking at six lines of a Shakespeare sonnet or a single paragraph from one of Jane Austen's novels. Our teacher had been trained in the golden age of English studies at Cambridge. He was influenced by some seminal books about how to read literature carefully. These included *Practical Criticism* by the literary scholar I.A. Richards. Books like these showed that any single line of great writing could be mined to great depths for complex meaning and insights into human life. Their writers believed that understanding literature wasn't about gaining a fuzzy impression of what the author might have meant, and wasn't like a visit to a historical theme park. It was a combined intellectual, emotional and moral enterprise to discover what the greatest minds of the past were trying to convey. It was akin to the reverent attention that previous generations applied to the Greek and Roman classics, and followers of the world's main religions still bring to their scriptures.

In recent years, a number of people have proposed that literary studies should form part of the curriculum in medicine as well, either at medical school or in postgraduate training. Some have even set these up within programmes for teaching medical humanities. Others have done so as free-standing ventures, driven by their own individual passion. In New York, Rita Charon – a hospital physician and a literary scholar in her own right – runs a Masters' course in narrative medicine at Columbia University. Its aims include enriching students' skills in close reading and literary analysis. In London, the GP John Salinsky has for many years encouraged trainees in general practice to read great novels, as well as taking them on visits to the theatre during their specialty training. These projects are based on the belief that literature can help doctors learn important truths about the human condition and increase their compassion at work. More specifically, they draw on the idea that if you learn to read a written text properly, you may become more expert in concentrating on the words that patients say as well. It can transform your understanding of what it means to listen, *really* to listen, to what patients have to say.

There is a standard medical way of listening, but there is also a deeper and more human way of listening that is in fact remarkably similar to studying a line in a poem or a sentence in a novel. For example, if a patient says 'this bunion is driving me to despair' the routine medical response is to look at the bunion. But why exactly has the patient chosen the word 'despair', and what does that signify? If we develop the art of attentive listening, and follow this up with the right question, this apparently random word may open up a far more elaborate story, steeped in personal meaning: 'I slept badly last night because I was so worried about my job interview, then on my way to my job interview I was so distracted that I tripped over my bunion, was in agony, made a mess of the interview, my husband is furious because we need the money, I don't know how much longer I can cope...'

JOHN LAUNER

Although we often choose to listen to only the 'thinner' version of such a story, we know – at least in principle – how important it is to try and engage with the 'thicker' one. It makes an enormous difference to the relationship with the patient, the quality of the encounter, the kind of treatment decision that is reached, the likelihood that the physician's recommendations will be followed and the clinical outcome improved. The risks of a failure to pay attention to the words go beyond mere misdiagnosis or poor concordance with treatment: they encompass what the sociologist Arthur Frank has called 'misrecognition', a fundamental failure to engage with what patients have come about, and who they are. They also include the risk of letting the story remain 'stuck'. Without active listening, and attentive questioning, the patient's story may remain the same as it always was, rather than evolving into something more creative and more helpful.

I have always been attracted to the idea of teaching doctors how to do close textual reading, and on a few occasions I have been able to put this into practice at residential workshops for GP trainers. Each time I have chosen two poems for them to study. The first is 'The Collar' by the seventeenth-century priest George Herbert. It describes his struggle with his religious vocation: the 'collar' in the title refers to his clerical neckwear but also to the yoke he felt his role imposed on him. The other poem is 'The Building' by Philip Larkin – one of the most acerbic but evocative poets of more recent years. The 'building' is a large general hospital. In the course of the poem, Larkin draws his readers into it, following human beings from the waiting room into their appointments and onto the wards, from where they may or may not ever return to their normal lives:

> Humans, caught
> On ground curiously neutral, homes and names
> Suddenly in abeyance; some are young,
> Some old, but most at that vague age that claims
> The end of choice, the last of hope; and all
> Here to confess that something has gone wrong.

Neither of these poems is straightforward. Both contain words and phrases that are unfamiliar, or used in unusual ways, particularly the case with the older poem. The first effect of reading them is to slow the reader down, not just from the ordinary pace of life but from the usual speed of reading as well. Each poem has its own rhythm – choppy and agitated in Herbert's poem, lilting and hypnotic in Larkin's, thus creating entirely different emotional responses. They aren't short poems either. 'The Collar' is around a whole page long, 'The Building' around twice that length. They require sustained concentration, not just the brief glance one might give to an email.

When I studied them with the GP groups, we needed every moment of the two hours we had assigned to the exercise. What we got out of it in consequence was very rich. Some of the doctors present were deeply moved by Herbert's confession of inner turmoil, and it helped them express similar feelings in them in relation to their own work. Others said that Larkin's account of a medical institution helped them to see these through different eyes. Many of them said it was the first time they had understood why close reading of difficult poetry was worthwhile, or that they were capable of doing so.

Would workshops like this make a difference to the way that doctors practise, or improve the care of their patients? In previous generations, educated people would have assumed that the answer was yes. In terms of today's standards of evidence-based training, it might be harder to prove such a claim. Yet it makes intuitive sense. Learning this kind of linguistic attentiveness cannot possibly do any harm to doctors and their patients. Learning that words are important, and studying them with care, are parts of a rounded education in any subject. In medicine, close reading may matter in fact more than anywhere else.

43

MEET YOUR MICROBIOME

....

Some time ago I had the privilege of meeting Elling Ulvestad, a Norwegian microbiologist who is also a philosopher. He is a man of tremendous warmth and energy, as well as having inexhaustible enthusiasm for his subject. It takes little time for him to convince anybody that the world is in great need of a philosophy that is properly informed by microbiology, not to mention the other way around. Here are the kinds of facts that Professor Ulvestad has on the tip of his tongue. First, we carry ten times as many bacterial cells around on our bodies as we do of our own cells (microbes are very much smaller than our own cells, which is why this is possible). If you also count the viruses that inhabit bacteria – known as bacteriophages – the ratio of microbes to human cells on each of us is probably more like 1000:1. Next, although we commonly regard bacteria as enemies, only around a hundred species regularly infect human beings, while literally millions of others either ignore us or co-operate with us in ways that would make our survival impossible without them. We are, in other words, not isolated individuals but walking ecologies. Our lumbering, multi-cellular bodies act as unwitting landlords to a vast community of far more resilient lodgers who could happily move to alternative accommodation in someone else's gut or skin – and quite often do.

Ulvestad's understanding of the interaction between humans and microbes goes far beyond numbers. He points out that microbes have been the 'chief molecular innovators' of the biological world. Evolution has been built on microbes' ability to develop, combine, or incorporate themselves into more complex forms. For a start they are, quite literally, our ancestors – with all modern life forms being their different descendants. They have also managed to become absorbed within our own DNA. Forty-five per cent of human DNA consists of sequences derived from microbes that are not only able to copy themselves during reproduction but also to move around within our chromosomes. The mitochondria that produce all the energy in our cells are themselves the descendants of formerly free-living bacteria. Although they have lost the ability to reproduce independently, they have compensated by managing to shield themselves from destruction by the human immune system.

Our intestines, immune systems and even our brains are dependent on their resident bacteria. For example, if laboratory mice are raised with intestines entirely free of germs, they behave differently from mice living in natural environments who automatically pick up friendly bacteria. If those laboratory mice are allowed to pick up bacteria while still in infancy, their behaviour becomes normal. If they are already adults, their behaviour remains abnormal: in other words, it is too late for the bacteria to help them with their own development. As Ulvestad argues, development 'ties the organism up in a system of references to other living and non-living entities'. Immunity from disease, he points out, is more than a simple matter of one organism fighting off another. Instead, he argues, it should be understood as 'a relational property that transcends the boundary of the organism'. It should not surprise us if eradicating a germ like *Helicobacter pylori* from the stomach (because it can cause ulcers) may result in a microbial backlash with a possibly increased incidence of asthma, along with diabetes and other medical problems.

Humans are sometimes held up as the ultimate example of the ability to transfer information from one generation to the next, through the use of language and culture. However, bacteria are equally adept at social learning. They transfer some of their genes between each other with massive frequency, so that in some of their species only about forty per cent of the DNA is common to all individuals. Ulvestad describes how they are able to take up ready-made genes from a mobile gene pool, and he likens this to the rapid uptake of new ideas by humans of information from the internet. This can sometimes be to the disadvantage of humans, for instance in the way that the germ causing gonorrhoea has developed resistance to all known drugs. It can also benefit us. One example is the way that the Japanese people who regularly eat seaweed can digest a sugar called porphyran because the bacteria on seaweed can transfer their gene for the appropriate digestive enzyme to the bacteria who live in the human intestine, making it possible for them to do the digestion on our behalf.

Bacteria also indulge in what Ulvestad calls 'cross-talk': they release and sense molecules that allow them to respond to the environment in a co-ordinated manner – for example by manufacturing protective films around themselves as a group, to defend against antibiotics. They often do so by a process known as 'quorum sensing': this enables them to know when their numbers are sufficient for such collaborative projects to be feasible.

One of Ulvestad's missions is to try to help everyone move away from the 'war' metaphor when talking about microbes (as in headlines like 'doctors defeat invasion of deadly bugs'). This pervasive metaphor in medicine arose in the nineteenth century, largely because most researchers were doctors, and they focused almost exclusively on the bacteria that cause diseases. He reminds us that at least one of the great early immunologists – the Russian, Ilya Mechnikov – was more concerned with studying how competition and co-operation were finely balanced in biology. More than a century after Mechnikov, this perspective has become almost universal in evolutionary and biological studies. A modern evolutionary view does not see any organisms – from viruses to humans – as intrinsically good or bad, but applies scientific curiosity in order to establish how hosts and infectious agents negotiate relationships along a scale from lethal hostility to symbiotic harmony. Ulvestad writes: 'As scientists, we need to acknowledge the fact that we are only studying a brief interlude of biological time, which represents the current trade-offs reached by contemporary organisms subject to a number of evolutionary forces... These forces are still acting to diversify and complicate the biological processes, and the results of the trade-offs reached will be the challenges encountered by future scientists.'

If Ulvestad is right, the view that doctors often have of themselves as heroic warriors has surely run its course. We need to start thinking about infectious diseases, and maybe all diseases, not in terms of the battlefield but in the kind of mature, ecologically informed view that he sets out. A hopeful development in this respect in the Human Microbiome Project, which aims to identify all the groups of microbes on the human body, and to analyse their roles in health human functioning and development. Many of our health-giving microbes have never been isolated or grown in laboratories before. One outcome of this project has been to establish that that there is a remarkable diversity of organisms among healthy people, with each of us bearing a relatively unique 'microbiome' alongside our unique genome. While some microbiomes may turn out to be associated with particular diseases or syndromes, others may confer protection.

Every generation of doctors and scientists is inclined to regard itself as having reached a pinnacle of understanding. We incline rather easily to the belief that our overall framework for understanding the world has been perfected, and it is only the details that remain to be filled in. Ulvestad's view has the potential to shake this complacency for the next generation of medical researchers and clinicians. If the last fifty years has been the age of the genome, we may be about to enter the era of the microbiome, when we start to pay respect not only to ourselves, but also to the far more ancient, numerous, adaptable and largely collaborative microbes on which our existence depends.

44

OPIUM

....

I once carried out a morning clinic where the first two patients both requested opiates but for entirely different reasons. The first patient was an elderly man with bone cancer. He came for a repeat prescription for a concentrated morphine solution to control his pain. I readily gave him what he asked for. The next patient was a young woman who said she was visiting from Glasgow and told me she was recovering from heroin addiction and was on a withdrawal programme there. She told me a story of having had her handbag stolen the previous day with her prescription in it, and needing a replacement. I politely refused. She left with little protest. A visitor from another planet, observing these two consultations, might have been puzzled as to why I was so generous with one person, and so strict with the other. I would have had to explain that, sadly, consultations like the second one are about twenty times as common as the first in inner city practices: the first patient's request was entirely legitimate, while the second was almost certainly deceitful, and driven by a craving for the drug itself. Almost every GP will prescribe in these circumstances only to patients they know, or at the request of a doctor elsewhere who does.

For patients and doctors alike, opiates are a blessing and a curse, a source of angelic relief from suffering and a diabolical cause of it. Morphine and heroin draw their users into the same polarised identities as the drugs themselves. We admire one group as moral heroes for taking these as they face the ultimate challenge of their lives. We approach the other group too often as moral failures – with suspicion at best, rejection at worst. No other class of drugs has such powerful physical and psychological effects. None has such a Manichean image in our society, culture or political debates.

It is tempting to believe that this is a relatively recent state of affairs, but it is not. A book called simply *Opium*, by the chemical pathologist Tom Dormandy, examines these drugs from every conceivable angle. Dormandy died recently at the age of eighty-six. He was a polymath and linguist who took his basic medical exams three times over – in Rumania, Switzerland and London – each time political circumstances in the 1940s forced him to move. He had previously published books on tuberculosis and art history, as well as being an accomplished painter. In *Opium* he displays a comfortable, almost affable familiarity with multiple languages and cultures, world history, politics and literature, as well as pharmacology.

The opium poppy, Dormandy explains, is ancient and ubiquitous. Lake dwellers in Switzerland consumed its seeds in buns in the late Stone Age. In Egypt and Mesopotamia, physicians prescribed poppy juice along with prayers, incantations, amulets and religious rites. Homer described how Helen of Troy added it to wine to cheer up her guests. The Roman emperor Nero succeeded to the throne after his mother had used it to dispose of his rivals. During barbarian times, opium disappeared from Western Europe but reappeared in Baghdad. In AD 1130 the physician Abulrayan al-Biruni noted that some pilgrims to Mecca sometimes took fatal overdoses. He enumerated the ten basic symptoms of overdose: 'lethargy, lockjaw, uncontrollable itching, watering eyes, paralysis of the tongue, discoloured extremities and nails, profuse cold perspiration, painful but ineffective vomiting, convulsions and death'. As Dormandy notes, 'little could be added to the list today'. In later centuries, opium cultivation moved between continents. Under the Ottoman Empire, the poppy fields in Turkey spread for hundreds of miles. In the eighteenth century, production moved to the Ganges valley, where the plantations were controlled by local potentates until the British colonists took them over. In the twentieth century, cultivation was concentrated in the 'Golden Triangle' in northern Thailand, and later in Afghanistan.

Some of the facts about opium covered in the book are well known. It played a prominent part in the Romantic movement, particularly for the poet Coleridge and his contemporary Thomas de Quincey. Opium derivatives and synthetic substitutes – including heroin itself – had originally been marketed as 'harmless' substitutes. The pioneer of palliative care, Dame Cicely Saunders, first promoted effective doses of opiates for terminal cancer, and introduced hospices where this could be practised. However, for every page of this book that covers such familiar ground, I found fifty that introduced me to new information. Some of this comes as a shock. In Victorian times, for example, opium consumption was almost universal in England. It was sold as a soothing medicine for babies, and added to beer for to farm workers. In the First World War, a large number of fighters in the trenches were sustained by opium. When the French Army mutinied in 1917, it was directly because supplies of morphine were withheld from the troops.

Dormandy's unflinching coverage of war and its relation to opium is among the great strengths of his book. In a chapter entitled 'The most wicked of wars', he gives an account of a singularly cynical campaign carried out by the British Empire. This was the destruction of China as a viable state in the mid-nineteenth century in two wars fought for the explicit purpose of sustaining profits and tax revenue through opium sales by British companies. In the course of these 'opium wars', the British army razed and looted the emperor's summer palace in Beijing. It had been one of the wonders of the world – a city in itself, containing lakes, mock mountains, gorges, bridges, a botanical garden and a zoo. It was also the repository of three thousand years of international arts and crafts including ceramics, carpets, textiles, furniture, paintings, gold ingots, bronzes, precious stones and an incomparable library. Its destruction would have been the equivalent of burning down Kensington Palace, the Victoria and Albert Museum, Buckingham Palace, the British Museum and everything in between, as a punitive measure. The sacking of the summer palace, and the massacres that accompanied it to preserve the British opium industry, still affect Chinese perceptions of the west to this day. Dormandy points out how ironic it was that the Chinese victims of these events became characterised as 'the yellow peril' for later bringing their addictions, and their opium, to the United States. He also describes how thousands died on the journey there, on what were effectively slave ships, or perished later in the gold mines of California.

Looking at more recent events, *Opium* examines the part played by the drug in the Vietnam War and the interminable conflict between the western powers and Afghanistan. Almost from the start of the ten-year conflict in Vietnam, 'opium and its derivatives were the props of increasingly venal regimes in Saigon'. Working together with Corsican gangsters, the Central Intelligence Agency provided armed back-up for supplies to the native market and the US army. By 1972, eighty-five per cent of soldiers were being offered heroin within a day of arrival, and thirty-seven thousand were addicts. Trade was open and supervised by the President's intelligence chief. GIs sent large lumps of heroin back home, sometimes buried in the wounds of a corpse in a body bag due for repatriation. Dormandy presents a scarcely more reassuring picture of the current state of affairs in Afghanistan, which he characterises as 'a twenty-first century narco-state'. In the 1970s, the country produced 700 hundred tonnes of opium a year. After the Russian invasion destroyed peacetime agriculture, this rose to 4,600 tonnes. When the Taliban defeated the Russians with US support, this dropped back again to 185 tonnes, but since the US reversed its support for the Taliban and staged its own invasion, it has risen to record levels. In 2010, around eighty per cent of the Afghan police and sixty per cent of the army were reckoned to be on the take.

Dormandy offers no easy solutions for anything – from the clinical challenges of addiction to the repeated eruptions through recent history of opium-fuelled wars. Yet while admitting it was impossible for him to end the book on an upbeat note, he argues that unmitigated gloom would be unjustified, especially as bio-technology is making the opium fields redundant. I hope he is right, but so far it looks unlikely. Currently, opiate use is increasing uncontrollably. Patients who use them to satisfy their craving vastly outnumber those requesting them from physicians for pain relief alone. In the United States and Canada, deaths from overdoses of opiates, whether natural or synthetic, prescribed or otherwise, have become a major epidemic. Dormandy's hope that 'the less bad may be allowed to replace the bad' could take a long time to materialise.

45

MEDICINE AS POETRY

....

Before I studied medicine, I did an English degree. It was at a time when cultural studies had not been invented and close reading of literary texts was still in fashion. There were a few books on this topic that were considered to be classics, and one of them was by a writer called William Empson. It had the title *Seven Types of Ambiguity*. Empson was something of a legend because he had come up to Cambridge to study mathematics in the 1920s but changed to English literature, wrote the book aged twenty-one while still an undergraduate, and was then expelled without a degree after a servant found condoms in his college room. He subsequently became a scholar of Chinese literature and a poet of distinction in his own right, while leading a colourful personal life. The reason his book became a classic was because of the way he argued that great poetry depended not just on its capacity to express complex meaning but on its ability to convey several different meanings at the same time.

The seven types of ambiguity that Empson describes in his book are not exhaustive. Rather, they represent points along a scale. At one end of this scale are straightforward devices like the use of metaphor, which is almost universal in poetry, and simply calls to mind an interesting comparison (for example, 'I wandered lonely as a cloud'). At the other end of the scale, there is the kind of writing that leaves readers having to make up their own minds entirely about what the author really means. The best known example of this is probably a novel by Henry James called *The Turn of the Screw*, where a children's governess describes events that are might be either real or imagined, and the author never resolves this uncertainty. In between, Empson describes a range of other types of ambiguity. These include the striking use of opposites, word play, revealing slips of the pen, meanings that seem to have emerged in the writer's own mind during the process of writing, and unclear expressions that leave the reader to fill in the gaps.

Since changing to medicine, I have always taken an interest in the use of language in the consultation. However, I had more or less forgotten about William Empson and his book until I recently came across a reference to it in an unexpected context − an essay on medical ethics by the Australian physician Paul Komesaroff. In contrast to almost everything ever written about communication skills, Komesaroff argues that ambiguity in medical conversations can be a valuable source of understanding. While scientists usually seek certainty, clarity and the elimination of divergent meaning, he suggests, medical communication often requires 'the deliberate preservation of uncertainty'. Drawing on Empson and others. including the philosopher Emmanuel Levinas, Komesaroff puts the case for respecting ambiguity in our use of language. 'We rely on ambiguity', he writes, 'when we need to express new meanings, when we wish to give voice to new or difficult ideas: for example, when we are trying to discern the goals of treatment or to clarify an emotional response.'

Komesaroff is not arguing in favour of muddled expression or miscommunication. Instead, he sets out a more profound and sophisticated view of the nature of language than the one that dominates medical thinking, where one word or phrase is generally believed to represent only a single thing or idea. He points out how all effective communication has to start with a suspension of presuppositions, and a search for a way 'to break through the curtain of mutual uninitelligibility'. This means opening oneself to 'suggestiveness and allusiveness'. It involves the careful, tentative use of 'the same devices, rhetorical forms, figures and tropes generally eschewed by philosophers and scientists, but embraced by poets and creative writers'. Speech, he reminds us, 'is not a solitary or impersonal exercise or a thought, it is not a process of mediation among contested propositions; it is a shared adventure of creation and discovery'.

Reading Komesaroff, and recalling the book by Empson after all these years, brought to mind some occasions when my interactions with patients succeeded not because of medical knowledge, but through subtle exchanges of language of the kind that both writers are describing. For example, I remember a patient who came in saying: 'There are three things I want to see you about.' Something about her emphasis on the word 'three' led me to ask immediately: 'What's the fourth?' She told me. It was the most important problem on her mind, and we never needed to return to the others. Another patient, irate at something I had said to challenge him, called me a 'fat lot of use' and stormed out of the room. His comment drew my attention to the fact I was overweight at the time, but it turned out to be accurate in other ways as well. Two weeks later, he returned to say he had thought about what I said and decided it was true and useful. More recently, a patient came to see me with a chronic skin condition, saying she felt like Job in the Bible, who was afflicted with incurable boils. I asked why she chose that comparison, and she listed a catalogue of disasters in her life recently, including the loss of her job and home. We were then able to discuss how the Book of Job ends, with its hero restored to health and prosperity, and how 'the Lord blessed the latter end of Job more than his beginning'.

Such consultations do not take place every day – although elements of them may be present more often than we suspect. As Komesaroff suggests, they can happen at critical moments, or when the mismatch between the language brought by the patient and the standard one offered by doctors is so great that we are compelled to explore radical alternatives. I never kept a diary of such exchanges over the years, but now wish I had done so. I would certainly encourage students and trainees to look out for the times they go beyond the banal formulas of everyday medical conversations and find themselves moving into similes, metaphors, allusions, puns, humour, paradox or other imaginative forms of speech. If they did so, they would discover that medicine can be poetic, in the true meaning of the word.

46

THE BREATHTAKINGLY SIMPLE FACTS OF LIFE

....

How much oxygen do you consume in a day? If you calculate it (the proportion of oxygen in the air, times the volume of one breath, times your breathing rate, times minutes per day) it comes to around five hundred litres per day. We are largely unaware that we consume so much gas, probably because we cannot see or feel it, except when a gust of wind blows on our faces. We are of course far more aware of how much food we consume, because we can detect it with every one of our senses. It totals around six hundred grams per day for the average healthy person. These gaseous and solid fuels enter our bodies by different and parallel tubes, but they end up interacting with each other in the same way as in any other internal combustion engine, with the release of energy and production of waste products along the way.

Essentially, the purpose of all this energy is self-replication. Living forms first evolved from inanimate objects – probably through chemical reactions in rocks – in order to manufacture replicas or near-replicas of themselves. Everything that they (and *we*) have done ever since has been directed towards the same result. Genes use energy to reproduce genes, cells use it to manufacture other cells, organisms use it to perpetuate their own kind, and families or groups use it to look after each other. We are in effect internal combustion engines dedicated to the production of identical or similar ones. This is somewhat alien to our everyday thinking, even as doctors. Most of us never feel subjectively that our own lives are driven by such very basic principles. An orthopaedic surgeon who is replacing someone's hip on the operating table, for example, is unlikely to be thinking about how the patient is burning up carbohydrates to stay alive, or how the operation might contribute to the preservation of the species by sustaining a productive member of the community. If we do try to think in this way, we may suffer the kind of existential discomfort that leads some religious believers to dismiss these ideas as the work of the devil. Even without this denial, we may still feel that these facts, and the connection between them, are of no practical use in the day-to-day pursuit of medical work.

Such a view would be wrong. A remarkable consensus has now emerged in biology that the living world can effectively be understood in exactly these terms, and that there is much to be gained by doing so. According to this point of view, our lives basically involve trying to apply energy from oxidation in the most efficient way possible, for the purpose of producing or supporting progeny and kin. In the words of biologist Bobbi Low: 'All living organisms have evolved to seek and use resources to enhance their reproductive success. They strive for matings, invest in children or help other genetic relatives, and build genetically profitable relationships. In biology, this is not a controversial proposition, and it follows that organisms will act as though they are able to calculate costs and benefits.'

Broken down into its constituent parts, this makes a lot of sense. All of our activities – procreation, raising children and grandchildren, making homes, building communities, forming alliances and fighting with enemies – can be seen as different contributions to the same simple purpose that living organisms have pursued since life first started. A whole range of disciplines from psychology to anthropology are now using this approach to make sense of the world around us. Social scientists are applying it to look at how societies choose different forms of child-rearing, or relationships between the sexes, in order to adjust to the scarcity or abundance of resources around them. Neuroscientists are using it to examine how emotions operate – our best way of assessing our interactions with others and the environment, and of judging how far these are progressing our direct and indirect reproductive interests. Thus desire, affection, anxiety, envy and rage may each signal perceptions of opportunity or threat, and lead to different ways of investing energy. On this basis, you can understand all the choices we make in our everyday lives as pragmatic calculations, at either a conscious or unconscious level, about what we should do in order to bring about the best prospects for ourselves, our kin and our group.

Such a unified biological view does not depend on seeing the world as purely competitive. It can also help us to understand why people support the interests of their family or group collaboratively, through such things as philanthropy, culture, art, religion and law. Nor is such a view deterministic. It offers an over-arching explanation for human behaviour, but without excluding more immediate ways of understanding the world, ranging from molecular explanations to political ones. Each of these different levels of understanding can add layers of description or meaning to the others. However, when all is said and done, the basis of life remains the same. In scientific terms, it all comes down to respiration leading to replication. The facts of life are indeed breathtakingly simple.

47

MONKEY BUSINESS

....

I am probably not the first person to have wondered if human beings are so close to some of the other great apes, including chimpanzees, that a mad scientist somewhere might secretly have tried to create a hybrid. It was only recently that I discovered such experiments did indeed take place. They were led by a scientist who, far from being mad, was one of the mainstream researchers of his time. They were also carried out without any secrecy at all. As it turns out, the story also has a lot to teach us about the political nature of scientific research and its driving forces. The project took place in the Soviet Union in the 1920s, with lavish funding, a fanfare of international publicity, and support from the United States, France and elsewhere. The man who led the hybridisation experiments was a Russian professor of zoology called Ilya Ivanov. He had already become famous earlier in his career for perfecting the technique of artificial insemination in horses, as well as producing hybrids between a donkey and a zebra, a bison and a cow, and various kinds of rodents.

In 1910 Ivanov gave a presentation to the World Congress of Zoologists in Graz in Austria, proposing that it should also be possible to produce a hybrid between a human and one of the great apes by using the same technique. After the

Russian Revolution of 1917, his idea attracted interest from the new Bolshevik government. By 1924, he had obtained the enormous sum of $10,000 dollars to fund an expedition to Africa to catch chimpanzees and start his insemination experiments. Ivanov's own motive appears to have been mainly one of scientific curiosity, although he proposed it to the government as a way of proving Darwin's theory of evolution, and therefore providing a conclusive justification for the atheism that lay at the heart of Soviet ideology. The Russian historian Alexander Etkind argues that the politicians who supported the scheme may have had other, more complex motives as well. Some Soviet leaders, including the radical politician Leon Trotsky, may have seen the mission as part of a futuristic project to produce the perfect 'new Soviet man', free of undesirable traits such as the wish to own property. Others may have had a more personal aim: to obtain a secure supply of ape glands for implantation into ageing humans – a treatment that was widely believed to lead to rejuvenation.

In the West, the plan received enthusiastic support from leaders of the Association for the Advancement of Atheism. One of their leaders, the American lawyer Howard England, proposed that chimpanzees should be crossed with white people, gorillas with black people, and gibbons with Jews. He considered that each of those apes must be the ancestor of these different races. Quoted in the *New York Times*, he suggested that it would be possible in this way, 'to produce the complete chain of specimens from the perfect anthropoid to the perfect man'. Although Ivanov himself does not seem to have had such precise ambitions for interbreeding, he had no moral qualms in some other respects. Setting up base in the French colony of Guinea, with the keen co-operation of the Pasteur

Institute, he began to impregnate female chimps with human sperm, possibly from his son. He initially intended to persuade local black women to accept payment in dollars for artificial insemination with chimpanzee sperm. When they failed to show any enthusiasm for the idea, he planned to do so without their consent, in the guise of gynaecological examination. In spite of Ivanov's angry protestations that bourgeois prejudice was obstructing science, the French governor and then the Soviet authorities forbade him from doing so.

Ivanov was not discouraged for long. He returned to the Soviet Union with twenty chimpanzees, although only four survived the journey. He set up a 'primatological nursery' in Abkhazia on the Black Sea, where he evidently found five women who were willing to consent to insemination voluntarily, as loyal communists and in the interests of science. The demise of the remaining chimpanzees, and Ivanov's failure to achieve a single conception using sperm from new arrivals, put an end to the project. Ivanov was arrested and exiled in 1930, probably for unrelated reasons, and died from a stroke not long afterwards. The primatological nursery survived for much longer, providing apes and monkeys for experiments in space in the 1960s. A friend of mine who worked for an American television company in Russia in 1979 tells me he was proudly shown some chimpanzees in the botanical gardens in Sukhumi that were said to be descendants of Ivanov's original apes. The nursery finally closed during the war with Georgia in 1992.

Ilya Ivanov's dream – or nightmare – may not have been so improbable, at least in scientific terms. The divergence of humans and chimpanzees from a common ancestor possibly took place in two distinct evolutionary stages, with interbreeding for over a million years before a definitive separation of the species took place. Humans have two fewer chromosomes than other great apes but, as Ivanov knew, there have been many successful hybrids created from different species of horses, where the variation in chromosome count can be far greater. Some of these equine hybrids even have been fertile for a further generation. With modern reproductive technology, including intra-cytoplasmic sperm injection, it is possible that all the scientific difficulties that Ivanov faced could be overcome.

Assuming that no one else has succeeded in doing this by clandestine means, the obstacles standing in the way are probably cultural beliefs rather than in science itself. Trotsky's dystopian vision of an engineered perfect citizen vanished with his own exile from the Soviet Union and subsequent assassination. The faith of Soviet leaders in monkey gland treatment became a focus for ridicule. The racist beliefs that underpinned the project have become abhorrent to most scientists, while concern for animal welfare would make the idea appalling in the eyes of many others nowadays. Nor does anyone think that experiments like this are necessary to prove Darwin right (although, ironically, Ivanov's failure is sometimes cited nowadays by creationists as proof that humans and the great apes were never related in the first place). Yet Ivanov's hybridisation project, and the assumptions that lay behind it, were in line with similar scientific projects that continued well into living memory, under both dictatorships and democracies. This happened in areas like eugenics, animal experimentation, drug trials in the developing world, and experiments infecting prisoners with lethal diseases.

Ivanov's work is also a reminder that there is rarely such a thing as 'pure' science. Politicians and the scientific community decide where to invest their time and money according to the values, assumptions and aspirations of the time. It is possible that future generations may look back at some of our own grandiose research endeavours – particularly those devoted to providing marginal benefits to wealthy people in the northern hemisphere and astronomical profits for a few corporations – and consider these just as distasteful as some earlier forms of scientific monkey business.

48

MEDICINE UNDER
CAPITALISM

....

For about ten years, I have carried out annual appraisals on
doctors working in general practice. I do this on a freelance
basis, not as part of my salaried work. When I started this,
I used to claim my fees from a man called Steve, in an office
at the local health authority. Now Steve is no longer there.
Nor is his job, nor his office, nor the authority. Nowadays, I
send my invoices to an agency a couple of hundred miles away
called 'Shared Business Services Payables'. When I write the
invoices, I have to use a 'supplier number', identifying myself
as a private business that supplies services to the National
Health Service. I also have to include my 'purchase order
number', confirming that the NHS has agreed to buy those
services. My contribution as an experienced doctor trained
to appraise colleagues has effectively been absorbed into the
same system that deals with the supply of X-ray machines,
hospital beds, or toilet rolls.

This change of my identity – from an individual professional
to a business – is no random event. It is one small part of
an intentionally designed change in the public services in
England. It reflects an ideological shift that has taken place
over the last couple of decades, in the name of the political and
economic movement known as neo-liberalism. A generation

ago, anyone in the health service who used terms like supplier, purchasers, providers, competition, market, profit, efficiency or output would have been regarded as exceedingly strange. Now it has become our everyday language. In England, and in many other countries, medicine has moved from a welfare model to a capitalist one. Private companies are taking over an increasing proportion of services, even if these are still branded as part of a public system. In keeping with this, the language of the welfare state has been replaced by one of commerce and capitalism. At times, it can even seem subversive to challenge this.

In a book entitled *Capitalist Realism*, the cultural commentator Mark Fisher has examined how this process has taken place. He suggests that, since the fall of communist regimes in the 1980s, capitalism has successfully come to present itself around the whole world as the only feasible political and economic system. He demonstrates how politicians, bureaucracies, education, books and movies all now speak with a single voice. It is a voice that says that everything, including medicine and education, should be run like a business. 'For most people under twenty in Europe and North America', he writes, the lack of alternatives to capitalism is no longer even an issue. Capitalism seamlessly occupies the horizons of the thinkable'. As a result, things that seemed impossible in the past – such as the privatisation of public services – are presented as natural and inevitable, while alternative models of society are rendered unimaginable. Alterations in language are a significant part of how this happens.

Fisher's critique of neo-liberalism has been influential, but another recent publication has been devastating in its analysis of modern capitalism and its effects. In 2014, the French economist Thomas Piketty leaped from relative academic obscurity to worldwide fame with his book *Capital in the Twenty-First Century*. His focus is on wealth inequality – the widening gap between the poorest in society and the ultra-rich. The facts of inequality are staggering. The top three per cent of families in the United States now hold double the wealth of all the poorest ninety per cent of their nation put together. One per cent of the world's population owns half its wealth. In theory, modern capitalism should have benefitted everyone by raising the standard of living across the board and providing incentives for enterprise. In practice, Piketty argues, this simply does not happen. He and his team have used data from two centuries and twenty countries to demonstrate that economies expand quite slowly, while the return on investments rises four or five times as fast. The gap between those who have wealth and those who do not is therefore continually widening. The winners of the game may claim that they have earned their fortunes and power legitimately, through taking risks and making sound business choices, but the losers are left with a diminishing share of income and wealth, and are increasingly depicted as failures and undeserving.

The pictures painted by both Fisher and Piketty are not cheerful ones. Fisher describes the demoralisation of young people who are unable to imagine earning any significant wealth during their lives, in a world where nothing else is seen as carrying any value. Piketty warns of the risk that a tiny elite of high-income and high-wealth individuals will capture the political process, threatening our democratic institutions and values. Both produce evidence of these developments. At the same time, they also point to remedies. In Fisher's view, it is a matter of raising people's consciousness and helping them to become aware that the discontent they feel with their lives is a symptom not of personal insecurity, but of dysfunction and false values in the society around them. Piketty argues that governments can and should intervene to correct the inevitable injustices of capitalism, through progressive taxes and other means of wealth distribution.

There is no particular reason why doctors and other health professionals should be taken up with these issues more than anyone else – except that the business model challenges some of the core values of medicine. In terms of language, the use of words like 'output' in the health service is not the same as using words like 'care': doing so creates a particular attitude to patients, turning them into objects instead of persons. Splitting up services for economic reasons leads to poor communication and the loss of teamwork. For example, receiving X-ray results from a call centre abroad, simply because this is cheaper, carries far greater risks to patient safety compared to discussing these with colleagues in the same hospital who know and understand the clinical context. Outsourcing health care to businesses may lead to poor performance or – if profits fall – to private companies deciding to pull out. Most important of all, the wealth inequality that comes with modern capitalism is not an incidental nuisance as far as medicine is concerned. It is one of the principal determinants of ill health. These developments are not inevitable. Challenging them at any level – whether as language, practice or policy – may in fact be a professional duty as much as a political choice.

49

MEMORIES OF THE
WORKHOUSE

....

I trained as a doctor at the Middlesex Hospital, close to the centre of London. When it was built in the eighteenth century, the Middlesex was on the very edge of the city, in open fields, but London swallowed it up and then extended a huge distance beyond. The hospital found itself close to the capital's main shopping streets and private medical consulting rooms. It became a leading national centre for patient care and for training. Then history had some more tricks to play on it. In the 1980s, all the medical schools in London were reorganised, and it was merged with University College Hospital, originally founded because the Middlesex had refused to allow its students onto the wards. In 2005, the Middlesex finally closed down. It was finally demolished to make way for a commercial development of shops and expensive apartments. Only the listed chapel – a fantastical Byzantine creation from the 1920s, with a marble interior and mosaics – has been left intact.

Some of my memories of training at the Middlesex are good, but others are not. Among the most uncomfortable ones are from the out-patient clinics. These took place not in the main hospital but in a drab brick building a hundred metres further north, in Cleveland Street. Patients sat massed together, all waiting in one large hall. The doctors sat at desks at the front of the hall, and saw each patient in full sight of everyone, and within earshot of the front rows. There was a distinctly 'poor law' feel about the place, as if patients should be grateful to be seen at all, even if their suffering was a public spectacle. Some of the doctors – although not all – had attitudes that reflected this. Once, in a side room off the main hall, I witnessed the most horrible consultation I can remember. In front of at least a dozen medical students, a famous surgeon broke the news to a middle-aged man that his cancer would require removal of half his face. With an ineptness that makes me wince to this day, he stuttered out a ghastly mixture of hints, euphemisms and evasions that forced the man to confront him in order to elicit the full horror of his disease. If I could have chosen one word to describe both the place and its proceedings, I probably would have used the word Dickensian.

The word would have been especially apt. Like many hospital buildings in London, the out-patient department had once been a workhouse. It was built around the same time as the Middlesex itself, to accommodate destitute parishioners from nearby Covent Garden. It expanded after the New Poor Law came into force in 1834, bringing in atrocious conditions of near-starvation and forced labour for the inmates. It carried on as a workhouse until the Middlesex purchased the building early in the twentieth century. However, what no one realised until very recently was that this was no ordinary workhouse. It was the one that Charles Dickens drew on for his best-known masterpiece, *Oliver Twist*.

When Dickens wrote his novel, he never identified the exact institution he had in mind. Historians knew that he had lived in this part of London in his early childhood, in somewhere called Norfolk Street, and that he had returned there in his late teens. By the twentieth century, no street with that name existed, so no one imagined that Norfolk Street was anywhere near Cleveland Street, or that Dickens might have been familiar with its workhouse. It was only in 2010, when the Middlesex Hospital had already been destroyed and the out-patient building was sentenced to the same fate, that local people started to look for a connection that might justify an appeal. They approached the historian Dr Ruth Richardson and asked if she could find something – anything – that might serve as evidence. With four weeks to go before the local council was due to make its final decision about demolition, Richardson pored over old maps of London. She then made a discovery so exciting that it made her 'yelp out loud with delight'. Norfolk Street wasn't simply nearby: it was the old name for the southern part of Cleveland Street, abutting the Middlesex Hospital. The young Charles Dickens and his family had lived nine doors away from the workhouse gates! Once Richardson had established that this was almost certainly the model for the workhouse in Oliver Twist, it was put on the list of protected buildings, although the fate of other parts of the site – including the Master's House, two receiving wards, some old Nightingale wards at the back, and the workhouse burial grounds – is still uncertain. They are now under threat of being lost beneath a tower block.

Following her discovery, Richardson published a book on Dickens, the workhouse, and the London poor. It brings the novelist and his times vividly to life. Dickens spent the formative years of his childhood walking past the portal of the Cleveland Street workhouse, with its stone relief exhorting passers-by to 'Avoid Idleness and Intemperance'. Later on, as a factory-boy in Covent Garden, he worked alongside young lads who would have been night-time inmates of the institution, farmed out as unpaid labour during the day. He may have heard from them how appalling life was there, with its notorious diet of thin gruel, reduced further during periods of punishment. When the Dickens family descended into penury, as they sometimes did, young Charles may well have been afraid that they would all end up there, with his parents separated from the children, and the siblings from each other, according to the regulations. Dickens may also have heard of other atrocities associated with the place. Just a few years before his family had moved to the area, a woman in labour was refused admission to the workhouse. She gave birth to her baby in the street outside. When the child died, the local people broke down the doors and carried the grieving mother into one of the workhouse wards.

In later life, Dickens became a passionate supporter of workhouse improvement. In 1866 he sent a donation to the great reforming doctor Joseph Rogers, physician to the Cleveland Street workhouse. Along with the donation, Dickens sent a note, saying that it was little wonder that 'the poor should creep into corners to die rather than fester and rot in such infamous places'. Rogers had already put his career on the line by protesting directly to Whitehall about the policy of putting women on a starvation diet for nine days after childbirth, to discourage others coming there for confinement. As a whistle-blower, having exposed serious neglect at the workhouse, he was later forced to resign. His campaigning efforts, along with the backing of eminent people such as Dickens, Florence Nightingale and the editor of *The Lancet*, Thomas Wakley, eventually led to the alleviation of conditions in the workhouses, and finally their abolition.

I cherish no nostalgia for the Cleveland Street workhouse building, or for what I saw there when it was part of the Middlesex, but I am glad it has been saved for posterity. It is a necessary reminder of the many different forms of cruelty that took place there and in similar institutions. Even more important, it stands as a testimony to those who stood up against that cruelty.

50

TAKING RISKS
SERIOUSLY

....

I was working with a group of Danish doctors on a course where they had a chance to talk about some of their most difficult patients: complex cases, challenging ones, people who had worn them down over the years by consulting very often but never getting any better. One theme came up again and again in their stories. It was the theme of risk. The doctors on the course didn't mean the kind of risks we spend so much time thinking about in medicine these days, such as blood pressure, smoking or obesity. What they had in mind was the way doctors sometimes take emotional risks with patients – for example by cracking a joke, being intentionally provocative, and even losing their temper. Time and again, they told stories of how they had turned the corner with patients they found difficult, not through being clever, but by showing their own emotions. The stories they told weren't about being punitive or moralistic. They were all about being authentic, being themselves.

Listening to them, I was struck by a certain paradox. I began to wonder whether we have become preoccupied in medicine with preventing health risks in patients, while forgetting the art of the taking emotional risks ourselves. To some extent this may simply be due to technology: we often spend more time nowadays looking at screens and writing requests for blood tests than we do talking with patients. But I suspect it may be part of change in our attitudes too. As doctors, we are more scared than we used to be of lawyers, managers, commissioners and regulators, and so we have become emotionally risk-averse. In the United Kingdom, I fear that the kind of courageous medicine my Danish colleagues were describing is becoming a thing of the past.

After hearing their own stories, I told the Danes about the most shocking – and possibly the most educational – consultation I have ever observed myself. It happened many years ago, when I was watching my own GP trainer at work in his surgery. He had already been there for many years, and he knew most of his patients extremely well. They also knew him as a charismatic man who looked them straight in the eye, laughed and cried with them without much inhibition, and almost invariably told them what he thought. The third or fourth patient of the day was a woman of about his own age, who greeted him by his first name as many of his patients did. She sat down and in a rather humdrum way she said she had a sore throat. Quick as a flash, my trainer asked her: 'And why the fuck have you really come?' I thought she would hit him, or walk straight out of the room to phone a lawyer. But she didn't. She answered the question instead – like a reflex, and without a moment to pause. Her real reason had nothing at all to do with a sore throat. Her doctor knew her well enough to realise this, and was brave enough to shock her into telling him what was really on her mind.

I have thought about this encounter many times over the years. What my trainer did on that occasion was outrageous, but it was also spontaneous, intuitive, and above all effective. I don't know whether he used the micro-second before he spoke to carry out a mental calculation about the risks he was taking and the likely benefits. I suspect not. However I am certain that he was working from a fundamental belief that what mattered most in medicine was doing whatever was going to help the patient most at that particular moment, and not any rules, guidelines, received wisdom, or any of the 'oughts' that generally dominate our conduct as doctors.

I have never been able to reproduce that precise example of risk-taking in a consultation, but it would be wrong even to try. Each of these transformational moments is by definition a one-off, suited only for that particular doctor and patient, and that consultation. But it is one of many incidents that has convinced me that the best medicine is often subversive. It doesn't always work through doing what is right and proper according to textbooks and governments. Sometimes it works instead by throwing all these things out of the window. It can even mean doing the diametric opposite of what you are 'meant' to do. (One doctor I know, for example, recently told a patient going through a family crisis that his drug habit probably reduced his anxiety and now was not the right time to try to give it up.)

This is an easy point to make, and most doctors with any experience would agree with it. The question is: how do we teach it? You clearly cannot go around telling medical students and junior doctors that it is fine to lose your temper, use four-letter words in the consulting room or advise patients to carry on taking addictive drugs. We need to impart the spirit of these experiences instead. The best way of doing this is probably by modelling it, and by demonstrating that if you take the right risks the earth won't open to swallow you up, and you won't be struck off either. But there are some sound general principles underlying good risk-taking, and it wouldn't do any harm to teach these far more than we do.

One principle is that evidence and medical guidelines may apply to groups of people, but they don't necessarily apply to individuals. The only place where evidence and individuals ever converge is through conversations, and every conversation is unique. Medical conversations can be dull and repetitive, but they don't need to be. They can also be creative, imaginative and enjoyable – and they probably need to be if they are to make any impact on patients. Another principle is that the contexts surrounding any medical conversation – including science, law, social rules and conventions – can influence an encounter, but they cannot substitute for it. If your heart tells you to break the relevant code, you may sometimes need to follow your heart. Indeed, it may be more ethical to do so than just to follow orders, as we know from innumerable examples of courage and risk-taking in the past.

Perhaps the most important principle behind courageous and effective risk-taking is that evidence and guidelines cannot be allowed to float around in a moral vacuum. In order to have meaning, they need to be embedded in a relationship and grounded in values. Taking emotional risks with patients, however scary, may be the best way of showing that relationships still matter in medicine.

51

THREE KINDS OF
REFLECTION

....

A few weeks ago I was invited to run a workshop on reflective practice at a conference. I assumed the arrangements would be much as usual – a ninety-minute slot with maybe ten or twelve people attending. I was mistaken. When I arrived I discovered the organisers had planned two slots for me, each lasting only three-quarters of an hour. Twenty-five people had already signed up for each of the slots. The thought of teaching reflective practice to such large numbers in such a short space of time seemed absurd, a contradiction in terms. It challenged my autonomic nervous system so much that I had to go to the toilet.

While there, I managed to collect my thoughts. I remembered how often health professionals complain that it's impossible to practise reflectively because time is so short and the circumstances too pressurised, and I wondered if I could use this opportunity to demonstrate the opposite: that reflective practice is *always* possible if you decide it's your main priority. I worked out a way to show exactly that.

I went to the seminar room where the workshops were taking place and arranged the chairs in a circle around the wall. I pushed the projector table and flip chart into a corner, and made sure I had no notes or papers in my hands or by my chair. Once everyone had come in and settled, I allowed a minute or two for people to sit in silence, expectantly. I introduced myself and pointed out that we had already created between us the ideal circumstances for reflective practice: a group of highly experienced professionals in a quiet room with no distractions and no interruptions. I told them that I didn't intend to teach them anything, but simply to allow them forty-five minutes of protected time for reflection with some clear structures and rules to make sure this happened.

Immediately, someone objected – in the nicest possible way. Since I was meant to be expert on the subject, she asked, couldn't I just explain to them how to make reflective practice happen in the impossible conditions of today's health service. I replied that this was exactly what I hoped to do, but through modelling it rather than telling people what to do. I told them that I was going to introduce a simple exercise that can be used almost anywhere, and that was going to demonstrate three different kinds of reflection. The first kind of reflection is inner dialogue: talking to oneself about a problem and what to do about it. The second kind consists of talking about this to another person. And the third kind involves having a further person (or persons) to witness the conversation and then offer their own thoughts about it.

Then I gave them the instructions for the exercise. First, I asked people to get into groups of three, trying if possible to get a mixture of individuals by gender, specialty or whatever. Next, I told each group to ask one person to think for a couple of minutes about a case or professional issue that was bugging them. I told them they should then allocate ten minutes for the person to talk about the problem, with one of the other two asking them questions about it – but nothing else. The role of the third person was just to listen to the conversation, keeping their own views and comments to themselves until the end. I told them that after eight or nine minutes of conversation the people in each group could briefly share their reflections about what had been discussed, but they should then rotate their roles straight away so that during the course of half an hour every member of each group got a chance to present a problem, ask questions or be an observer.

Even with such clear instructions, I knew from experience that conversations like this can turn into requests for advice. This calls forth a barrage of suggestions from everyone, so that no genuine exploration of the problem takes place. That may be fine in some everyday situations, but it isn't reflective practice. So I made things a bit harder for everyone by insisting that the questioners had to obey three simple rules:

1. You can only ask open questions (e.g. 'What have you thought of doing?' rather than 'Have you thought of discharging her?')

2. Every question must link up with words the case presenter has already used and not with your own ideas (e.g. 'What do you mean by "bad asthma?"' rather than 'Does the patient fit the criteria for home oxygen?')

3. You should withhold any suggestions or advice till the end, and avoid giving away your own thoughts by the way you ask your questions.

I've used variations of this exercise many times before but never under such pressure of time, or with a large group of people who were unknown to each other and had no previous training in this method. The outcome was very satisfying, both with this group and with the second group who followed them. Almost everyone reported being astonished by how hard it was to follow a strict set of conversational rules like this, and yet how rewarding the results were when they did. People taking on the role of questioners and observers said they were bursting to give advice and tell the case presenters exactly what they would do in their shoes – a habitual position of certainty and expertise that most doctors take on far too readily. Yet when forced to pay attention, withhold their own opinions, and only respond when enough time had passed for them to form a considered judgement, they were amazed at the quality of the reflections they were then able to share.

The commonest remark was that the case presenters' problems seemed to become resolved *through the very process* of talking, questioning and listening, and this seemed more productive than direct problem-solving of the kind that doctors do for most of the time.

Despite the simplicity of this exercise, it draws on a wide range of thinking about education, psychology and dialogue that are used in many other fields. Most people involved in educating professionals admire the work of Donald Schon and know about the distinction he made between 'reflection in action' (what one is able to do on the hoof by way of reflective practice) and 'reflection on action' (what happens afterwards). They will also be aware how much the quantity and quality of the latter, particularly if practised regularly, enhances the former. People may be less familiar with the ideas of thinkers like the Russian psychologist Lev Vygotsky and his contemporary, the linguist Mikhail Bakhtin. Although working in separate fields, they came up with theories to suggest that thinking, speaking and action are in essence not individual activities but ones that are formed through – and informed by – the social process of dialogue.

A similar approach is taken by 'systemic' psychotherapists, who work with clients mainly through the use of carefully crafted questions and dialogue rather than through advice and interpretation. These ideas all point towards a close interrelationship between the quality of the conversations we have with each other, the quality of reasoning that takes place within our own minds, and the quality of what we are then capable of producing as a result.

If the brief experience of these two short workshops is anything to go by, it shouldn't be hard to improve patient care through the three simple disciplines of focussing one's mind on an issue, having a proper dialogue about it with someone else, and then conferring with an independent witness to the dialogue. For that to happen, you first need to clear away the noisy paraphernalia that usually surrounds and distracts you, and insist that reflective practice comes first and makes a real difference. It isn't difficult, and it doesn't need to take long.

52

BRIEF ENCOUNTER

....

Sitting near the boarding gate with my family at an international airport, I noticed a young man and woman opposite me. Both were in their twenties. I assumed they were flying back home together to London at the end of their summer vacation. After several minutes neither had spoken and I realised they were strangers, although they looked as if they would make a suitable match. For a moment, I had the ridiculous thought of suggesting they should talk to each other. Such thoughts don't come into one's mind for no reason, and when the man got up to join the queue for the plane, I noticed the woman look up and follow him wistfully with her eyes. Seeing me watching her, she smiled slightly and blushed. I wondered if she would now try to stand behind him in line and strike up a conversation after all. However, by the time she joined the queue a large family had beaten her to it. There would be no conversation, nor the relationship that might have followed. I felt for the young woman. Most of us have no doubt been in the same position as her at some time – too shy to talk to someone we wanted to. But it also struck me what a good illustration the episode was of some fundamental principles of evolutionary psychology.

It was Darwin who first suggested that we should examine all human behaviour and feelings in the light of the drive for reproduction and the challenges it raises. No one took up his suggestion in any systematic way for a hundred years. However, the field of evolutionary psychology is finally coming into its own and beginning to equip us with the knowledge to 'read' encounters like this, and many others, just as we would with primates or other mammals. Drawing on the ideas of evolutionary scholars such as David Buss, Robin Dunbar and Christopher Boehm, I want to propose a way of deciphering the little mini-drama that I witnessed.

Homo sapiens, as Darwin realised, is no different from any other sexually reproducing species on the planet. Our overriding imperative is to reproduce – or to support our kinship group in doing so. If we want to make a direct contribution through having progeny ourselves, we need to do this during our years of maximum fertility, which for women happens to be during late adolescence and early adulthood. If it wasn't for the drive for reproduction, we wouldn't experience desire, and without desire the young woman at the airport would never have been interested in the man next to her.

Desire has to fix on the best available person at any given time and place. It is no use if you are in the arrivals area when a potential partner of the opposite sex is at the boarding gate. In that respect, you are no different from a wild flower that is never fertilised with pollen from a particular plant in a neighbouring field because the bee has flown off elsewhere. Outside romantic novels, very few people live their lives entirely free of desire until the one and only Mr or Ms Right comes on the scene. Our species would not have lasted very long if that had been the case. It is better to feel desire for someone who happens to cross your path – or whoever sits down in the chair next to you at the airport – rather than waiting for something that will never happen.

Having said that, desire is still highly selective. While on the alert for reproductive opportunities, everyone also instantaneously assesses others for their suitability as reproductive mates. This is presumably why the young woman in question was drawn instinctively towards the equally young and attractive man beside her rather than the considerably older grey-haired family man (myself) sitting opposite. She didn't need a checklist to work out that the younger man might fit a number of categories for a better match. In the same way, I intuitively recognised the two of them as a potential mating pair if not an actual one.

Desire is selective, but it is also contextual. As it happens, airports and other places of transit seem to be particularly good places to stimulate sexual attraction, for all sorts of reasons. Away from their familiar networks, people are deprived of the everyday comforts that might distract them from seeking a partner, but also free from the social judgements that might inhibit a liaison. It is no coincidence that stories of holiday romances and affairs with transient foreigners are so common.

In addition, desire is always accompanied by risk. It is in this area that evolutionary thinking may help us the most in deciphering the incident I witnessed. Although the young woman at the airport may have longed for the man to turn to her and engage in conversation, an intuitive assessment of risk seemingly led her to feel she couldn't take the initiative herself. As a woman, she was far from unusual in making this judgement – and for good reasons. Women carry far more risks to physical and personal safety than men do. These include not only the dangers of pregnancy and childbirth but also rejection, abuse, abandonment and worse. All of this is presumably why, across all cultures, it is hugely commoner for men of all ages and appearances to make sexual advances than for attractive young women to do so.

Perhaps the most interesting aspect of this episode was the unspoken communication that took place between the woman and myself. First there was that strange, almost telepathic contact that led me to have the weird fantasy of effecting an introduction between them. Such 'psychic' moments are not as bizarre as they may seem. We pick up people's intentions from the way they look and from their body language, and this in turn affects our thoughts without us even being aware this has happened, a process that some people call 'mentalisation'. As for her smile and blushing – a phenomenon that Darwin discovered is universal in our species, and unique to us alone – it disclosed her discomfort at having unwittingly displayed her private desires: something we simply aren't meant to do as we carry out our carefully concealed reproductive strategies.

Oddly, medical students are taught little or nothing about the theory of evolution. Most doctors will have read nothing about evolutionary psychology or may never even have heard of it. This is a great pity. As a framework for thinking about human interactions, it makes a good deal of sense. It is surprisingly simple and intrinsically fascinating. The airport episode shows its potential for understanding how we behave in everyday life, how we feel, and who we are.

53

POWER AND
POWERLESSNESS

....

Many years ago, I came up with an idea that every medical student should have to sign a special consent form when they started their training. The form would allow their medical school, at some random moment during the ensuing years, to admit them to hospital with an imaginary illness. According to this scheme, every student would suddenly receive a message out of the blue, saying that they had contracted severe pneumonia, a fracture of the hip or some other major condition. They would then be admitted to hospital and given more or less exactly the same treatment as if their assigned problems were genuine. Some might be put on intravenous drips and gastro-nasal feeds. Others might have limbs put in plaster casts. All of them would be confined to bed.

For some students, discharge after a week or two might be followed by having to move around on crutches or in a wheelchair for a further length of time – or even for the rest of their course. One or two might be obliged to simulate even worse disabilities: for example, being blindfolded for several weeks in order to experience the effects of a sudden loss of sight. There would be no appeal against these arrangements on the grounds that they were about to take their exams, go on holiday, or get married, or for any personal reasons. Just as in real life, they would have to accept the condition that had struck them down, and adjust to it.

My proposed scheme was of course entirely impractical, not to mention cruel and unethical. For that reason, I don't think I shared the idea with anyone else at the time. However its rationale was completely serious. It was to give all future doctors, at an early stage in their training, a realistic experience of what illness and hospital admission are actually like. They would learn how frustrating it can be to have one's life suddenly and catastrophically disrupted, and what it is like to be completely fit at one moment and then handicapped the next. It might teach them something else as well: how powerless patients can feel, not just because of their illnesses but because of what happens to them once they fall into the hands of the medical profession.

For hospital staff, admissions are just routine events, scarcely more dramatic than customers arriving in a shoe shop to buy a pair of shoes. For patients, by contrast, it represents a threefold loss of power. First there are the bodily symptoms themselves – the pain, breathlessness, immobility or whatever else brought them into hospital. Then there is the traumatic disruption of normal life, with all its comforting regularity and its assumed sense of control. But in addition there is a loss of power relative to the people who are looking after them, and to doctors in particular. For some patients, this aspect of their powerlessness is the worst.

As any patient will tell you, the power differential isn't just about doctors being well and patients being ill, or even about doctors being in the hospital voluntarily while patients are there on the whole without much choice. It is about the enormous range of privileges that any doctor – even the most junior – possesses by comparison with a person lying in a hospital bed. These include the privilege of standing up while the patient lies down, and of being dressed in normal clothes while the patient is in pyjamas. They include the rights of deciding if and when to come and talk to the patient, how much time to spend in doing so, and what to tell or not to tell. Each one of the unthinking everyday rituals of ward life carries with it a set of choices that are available to the doctor, while the patient can influence them either little or not at all.

There is another more pervasive aspect of doctors' power, although from inside the medical profession we may have little awareness of it. The French historian and philosopher, Michel Foucault, called it 'the medical gaze'. He used the term to describe the way we look at other people not as fellow humans, with subjective feelings and needs as rich as our own, but as objects of detached curiosity. He considered that this attitude wasn't an expression of scientific advance as we might believe. Instead, he regarded it as a distinctly political state of mind, linked to wider forms of oppression including economic and judicial ones.

When we doctors examine the surface of the body for evidence of disease, or poke into orifices to explore its interior, our overall purpose, according to Foucault, is to demonstrate and enact a particular kind of power. The way we do this, he argued, is an exact parallel to the way that the police, the tax authorities or other agents of the state exert power in their own different ways as well. Most doctors would probably find Foucault's thinking in this respect excessively harsh and one-sided. Perhaps it is, but it could account for much of the fear and alienation that patients feel when they come into contact with us. It could also help us to make sense of oppressive behaviour on the part of doctors, including widespread incivility, or the stigmatisation of certain patients including those on the social margins.

Arbitrary and compulsory admission to hospital is unlikely to find a place on the medical school curriculum, nor is Michel Foucault. However, there is a great deal doctors could do to sensitise ourselves, our students and our trainees to issues of power and powerlessness in medicine. When we take histories, we could inquire about the trauma of admission as well as its cause. We could ask not just *'where did the pain start?'* and *'what were you doing at the time?'*, but also *'what were you planning to do?'* and *'what is going to happen now that you can't?'* We could consider how our daily ceremonies – our ward rounds or clinics – can distance and humiliate patients in a hundred different ways instead of engaging them as equal partners. We could learn to use our speech and body language in ways that express a willingness to share power rather than imposing it.

As doctors, most of us probably don't think about our power as much as we should. Like people in any other job, we are preoccupied for much of the time by the constraints of our work: annoying regulations, irritating colleagues or managers, and shortages of time, money and other resources. Yet power over patients is constantly present in all our work. How we use or abuse this makes as much difference to them as our technical care.

54

FATHERS AND SONS

....

Oedipus, as everyone knows, inadvertently murdered his father and had sex with his mother. According to the story, he had not seen his parents since infancy, so he could not recognise the man he killed at the cross-roads, nor the queen whose city he saved from a plague, and whom he then married.

It is hard to know if people nowadays would be more familiar with this story than they are with any other Greek myth, had it not been for Freud. It was Freud – as everyone also knows – who believed that the story of Oedipus encapsulated a struggle that every child faces in its early years, as it tries to displace one parent in the sexual affections of the other.

Translated into developmental terms, the Oedipus complex makes a lot of sense. It is a kind of deadly serious dress rehearsal for the later business of finding the best available mate, while remaining realistic about the scale of the competition and the limits of one's own sexual power. In some ways, however, it is odd that Freud placed so much emphasis on the murderous impulses of small children rather than those of their parents. In the Oedipus story, it is actually the hero's father Laius who sets the tragedy in motion by believing a prediction that his son will one day kill him, and by issuing an order for the baby boy to be taken to the mountains and left there to die. The irony, of course, is that Oedipus survives to get his unwitting revenge – which fulfils the prophecy. In reality, parricides are vanishingly rare, whereas infanticides are sadly commonplace. It might be argued that we face a more precariously poised battle with our Laius complexes as parents than we ever did with our Oedipus complexes as children. Many parents would admit to having had to master feelings towards their offspring that were not far short of murderous at times. Even the most loving of parents will probably recall their first shocking awareness of being displaced by a ruthless, rebellious, self-willed infant with determined designs of its own – not on the marital bed, perhaps, but certainly directed at monopolising its parents' energies and investment.

If it is striking that Freud turned his attention to Oedipus rather than Laius, it is perhaps even odder that he did not concentrate on another story about a father with murderous intent towards his son: that of Abraham. It is a story with an altogether different outcome. Abraham, you may recall, follows a command from God to take his son, his only son whom he loves, to a place that God shows him, to sacrifice him there as a burnt offering. In a narrative of intolerable tension, we hear how Abraham takes his son up Mount Moriah, with a knife and wood for kindling, and binds him on an altar in order to butcher him. It is only at the last possible moment that an angel of the Lord stays Abraham's hand and points to a ram caught in a thicket as a sacrifice instead. (In the biblical passage the angel calls out to him, although in Rembrandt's famous depiction of this scene, the angel seizes Abraham's wrist, thus forcing him to drop the knife out of his hand.) The angel then blesses Abraham as a reward for passing this test of his faith. The correct name for the story is 'The Binding of

Isaac' but it is often referred to as 'The Sacrifice of Isaac'. The mistake may reflect many people's impression that Abraham's compliance with God's initial command is just as bad as if he had completed the act.

There are indeed many different ways of responding to the story. Many Jews, Christians and Muslims profess a straightforward admiration for Abraham's submission to God's will, regarding it either as exemplary in itself or because it demonstrates Abraham's utter trust that God will always do the right thing in the end. Most atheists, by contrast, are likely to see in the biblical text yet further proof of a vicious and arbitrary God who – if he existed – would deserve neither obedience nor respect. There is a subtler reading of the text than either of these. It was the reading favoured by some of the mediaeval Jewish commentators, who saw the resolution of the story as being implicit from the outset. This kind of symbolic understanding of stories, where time is collapsed and events are seen as synchronous rather than sequential, probably came more naturally to people before the Enlightenment than it does now. The nearest that we can get to such an understanding these days might be to say that the story is a narrative representation corresponding to our idea of ambivalence. In his heart, Abraham is torn between love for the son for whom he has always yearned, and his wish to destroy an heir who will one day supersede him. His struggle is both internal and external, with a God who is (to use theological language) both immanent and transcendent.

Many writers have understood that the story could have gone either way. There are ancient traditions that include the suggestion that Abraham really did slaughter Isaac. And in a more recent reconstruction of the story, the First World War poet Wilfred Owen described his own times in terms of an obdurate Abraham who had heard God's first, fatal command but then ignored its revocation:

> Behold,
> A ram, caught in a thicket by its horns;
> Offer the Ram of Pride instead of him.
> But the old man would not so, and slew his son.
> And half the seed of Europe, one by one.

As Owen realised, the drama of Abraham's struggle is an individual one but also a collective, and indeed a universal one. The choice between behaving like Laius or like Abraham is not a foregone conclusion at any time, or for any of us.

FURTHER READING

....

5. WHAT'S IN A NAME?

Winchester, S. (1999), The Surgeon of Crowthorne
   (London, Penguin).

10. ANNA O AND THE 'TALKING CURE'

Borch-Jacobsen, M. (1996), Remembering Anna O: A
   Century of Mystification (London, Routledge).
Breuer, J. [1895], 'Fräulein Anna O.' in S. Freud (1955),
   The Standard Edition of the Complete Psychological
   Works of Sigmund Freud, vol. 2, ed. J. Strachey
   (London, Hogarth Press).
Kaplan-Solms, K. & Solms, M. (2000), Clinical Studies in
   Neuro-Psychoanalysis (London, Karnac).

17. MYSTERIES OF THE MALE

Dawkins, R. (2004), The Ancestor's Tale: A Pilgrimage to
   the Dawn of Life (London, Weidenfeld & Nicholson).
Judson, O. (2002), Dr Tatiana's Sex Advice to All Creation:
   The Definitive Guide to the Evolutionary Biology of
   Sex (London, Chatto & Windus).
Kraemer, S. (2000), 'The fragile male', British Medical

Journal, vol. 321, pp. 1609–12.

Maynard Smith, J. (1978), The Evolution of Sex
(Cambridge, Cambridge University Press).

Ridley, M. (1993), The Red Queen: Sex and the Evolution
of Human Nature (London, Viking).

18. THE ENDURING ASYLUM

Wynne, C. (2006), The North Wales Hospital, Denbigh
1842–1995 / Ysbyty Gogledd Cymru, Dinbych 1842–
1995 (Rhyl, Gwasg Helygain).

21. THE PROBLEM WITH SEX

Appignanesi, L. & Forrester, J. (1992), *Freud's Women*
(London, Weidenfeld & Nicolson).

Carotenuto, A. (1982), *A Secret Symmetry: Sabina Spielrein
between Freud and Jung* (New York, Pantheon).

Covington, C. & Wharton, B. (eds.) (2003), *Sabina
Spielrein: Forgotten Pioneer of Psychoanalysis* (London,
Psychology Press).

Kerr, J. (1993), *A Most Dangerous Method: The Story of Jung,
Freud, and Sabina Spielrein* (New York, Alfred Knopf).

Launer, J. (2005), 'Mysteries of the male', *QJM*, vol. 98, pp.
919–20.

McGuire, W. (ed.) (1974), *The Freud/Jung Letters*
(Princeton, Princeton University Press).

Spielrein, S. [1912] (1994), 'Destruction as the cause of
coming into being', *Journal of Analytical Psychology*, vol.
39, pp. 155–86.

22. THE ART OF QUESTIONING

Tomm, K. (1988), 'Interventive interviewing: part III.
Intending to ask lineal, circular, strategic or reflexive
questions?', *Family Process*, vol. 27, pp. 1–15.

24. INTERPRETING ILLNESS

Bury, M. (2001), 'Illness narratives: fact or fiction?',
Sociology of Health and Illness, vol. 23, pp. 263–85.
Launer, J. (1978), 'Taking medical histories through
interpreters: practice in a Nigerian outpatient
department', *British Medical Journal*, vol. 2, pp. 934–5.
Mattingly, C. (1998), *Healing Dramas and Clinical Plots:
The Narrative Structure of Experience* (Cambridge
University Press, Cambridge).

26. YELLOW NOSE SIGN

Gabbay, J. (1982), 'Asthma attacked? Tactics for the
reconstruction of a disease concept', in T. Wright,
T. & A. Treacher (eds.), *The Problem of Medical
Knowledge: Examining the Social Construction of Medicine*
(Edinburgh, Edinburgh University Press).
Kuhn, T. (1970), *The Structure of Scientific Revolutions*
(Chicago IL, University of Chicago Press).
Strong, P.M. (1979), *The Ceremonial Order of the Clinic:
Parents, Doctors and Medical Bureaucracies* (London,
Routledge and Kegan Paul).

28. BREAKING THE NEWS

Candib, L. (2002), 'Truth telling and advance planning at the end of life: problems with autonomy in a multi-cultural world', *Families, Systems, and Health*, vol. 20, pp. 213–28.

Hudson Jones, A. (1998), 'Narrative in medical ethics', in T. Greenhalgh & B. Hurwitz (eds.), *Narrative Based Medicine: Dialogue and Discourse in Clinical Practice* (London, BMJ Books).

McCarthy, J. (2003), 'Principlism or narrative ethics: must we choose between them?', *Journal of Medical Ethics: Medical Humanities*, vol. 29, pp. 65–71.

33. ESCAPING THE LOOP

learning and communication', pp. 279–308 in *Steps to An Ecology of Mind* (Chicago IL, University of Chicago Press).

Oliver, C. (2004), 'Reflexive inquiry and the strange loop tool', *Human Systems*, vol. 15, pp. 127–40.

36. FOLK ILLNESS AND MEDICAL MODELS

Blumhagen, D. (1980), '"Hyper-Tension": a folk illness with a medical name', *Culture, Medicine and Psychiatry*, vol. 4, pp. 197–227.

37. THE FACTS OF DEATH

Clark, W.R. (1996), *Sex and the Origins of Death* (Oxford, Oxford University Press).

39. ON KINDNESS

Palmer, E. (2008), 'The kindness of strangers', *British Medical Journal*, vol. 337, p. 877.

Stacey, R.D. (2001), *Complex Responsive Processes in Organisations* (London, Routledge).

Suchman, A.L., Williamson, P.R., Litzelman, D.K., Frankel, R.M., Mossbarger, D.L., Inui, T.S. & the Relationship-Centred Care Initiative Discovery Team (2004), 'Toward an informal curriculum that teaches professionalism', *Journal of General Internal Medicine*, vol. 19, pp. 501–4.

40. CAPABLE BUT INSANE

Schreber, D.P. [1903] (2000), *Memoirs of My Nervous Illness* (New York NY, New York Review of Books).

41. ON THE RECORD

Aaslestad, P. (2009), *The Patient as Text: The Role of the Narrator in Psychiatric Notes, 1890–1990* (Abingdon, Radcliffe Publishing).

Macnaughton, R.J. & Evans, H.M. (2004), 'Medical

humanities and medical informatics: an uneasy alliance?
Is there a role for patients' voices in the modern care
record?', *Medical Humanities*, vol. 30, pp. 57–8.

42. CLOSE READINGS

Frank, A. (2001), 'Experiencing illness through
storytelling', in S. Tooms (ed.), *Handbook of
Phenomenology and Medicine* (New York NY, Springer).
Richards, I.A. (1929), *Practical Criticism* (London, Kegan
Paul).
Salinsky, J. (2001), *Medicine and Literature: The Doctor's
Companion to the Classics* (Abingdon, Radcliffe).

43. MEET YOUR MICROBIOME

Friedrich, M.J. (2013), 'Genomes of microbes inhabiting
the body offer clues to human health and disease',
Journal of the American Medical Association, vol. 309, pp.
1447–9.
Ulvestad, E. (2007), *Defending Life: The Nature of Host-
Parasite Relations* (Dordrecht, Springer).
Ulvestad, E. (2009), 'Co-operation and conflict in host-
microbe relations', *APMIS*, vol. 117, pp. 311–22.
Ulvestad, E. (2012), 'Psychoneuroimmunology: the
experiential dimension', *Methods in Molecular Biology*,
vol. 934, pp. 21–37.
Willyard, C. (2009) 'A tough controversy to stomach',
Nature Medicine, vol. 15, pp. 836–9.

44. OPIUM

Dormandy, T. (2012), *Opium* (New Haven CT, Yale University Press).

Lovell, J. (2011), *The Opium War* (London, Picador).

45. MEDICINE AS POETRY

Empson, W. (1930), *Seven Types of Ambiguity* (London, Chatto and Windus).

Komesaroff, P. (2005) 'Uses and misuses of ambiguity: uses of ambiguity', *Internal Medicine Journal*, vol. 35, pp. 632–3.

46. THE BREATHTAKINGLY SIMPLE FACTS OF LIFE

Chisholm, J. (1999), *Death, Hope and Sex: Steps to an Evolutionary Ecology of Mind and Morality* (Cambridge, Cambridge University Press).

Damasio, A. (1994), *Descartes' Error: Emotion, Reason and the Human Brain* (New York NY, Putnam).

Laland, K. & Brown, G. (2011), *Sense and Nonsense: Evolutionary Perspectives on Human Behavior*, 2nd edn (Oxford, Oxford University Press).

Lane, N. & Martin, F. (2012), 'The origin of membrane bioenergetics', *Cell*, vol. 151, pp. 1406–16.

Low, B.S. (2001), *Why Sex Matters: A Darwinian Look at Human Behavior* (Princeton NJ, Princeton University Press).

Nowak, R. (2011), *Supercooperators: Evolution, Altruism and*

Human Behaviour (London, Canongate).

Simpson, J. & Belsky, J. (2008), 'Attachment theory within a modern evolutionary framework', pp. 131–57 in J. Cassidy & P.R. Shaver (eds.), *Handbook of Attachment: Theory, Research and Clinical Applications*, 2nd edn (New York NY, Guilford Press).

47. MONKEY BUSINESS

Chandley, A.C., Short, R.V. & Allen, W.R. (1975), 'Cytogenetic studies of three equine hybrids', *Journal of Reproduction and Fertility*, vol. 23, pp. 356–70.

Bergman, J. (2009), 'Human-ape hybridization: a failed attempt to prove Darwinism', *Acts and Facts*, vol. 38, p. 12.

Etkind, A. (2008), 'Beyond eugenics: the forgotten scandal of hybridizing humans and apes', *Studies in the History and Philosophy of Biology and Biomedical Sciences*, vol. 39, pp. 205–10.

Patterson, N., Richter, D.J., Gnerre, S., Lander, E.S. & Reich, D. (2006), 'Genetic evidence for complex speciation of humans and chimpanzees', *Nature*, vol. 441, pp. 1103–8.

'Soviet backs plan to test evolution', *New York Times*, 17 June 1926, p. 2.

48. MEDICINE UNDER CAPITALISM

Fisher, M. (2009), *Capitalist Realism: Is There No Alternative?* (London, Zero Books).

Iacobucci, G. (2015), 'Outsourcing the NHS', *British Medical Journal* 350:875.

Marmot, M. & Wilkinson, R. (eds.) (2005), *Social Determinants of Health*, 2nd edn (Oxford, Oxford University Press).

Piketty, T. (2014), *Capital in the Twenty-First Century* (Harvard MA, Harvard University Press).

49. MEMORIES OF THE WORKHOUSE

Hurwitz, B. & Richardson, R. (1989), 'Joseph Rogers and the reform of workhouse medicine', British Medical Journal, vol. 299, pp. 1507–10.

Richardson, R. (2012), Dickens and the Workhouse: Oliver Twist and the London Poor (Oxford, Oxford University Press).

Richardson, R. (2013), 'Charles Dickens, The Lancet and Oliver Twist', Lancet, vol. 379, pp. 404–5.

50. TAKING RISKS SERIOUSLY

Charon, R. & Wyer, P. for the NEBM working group (2008), 'Narrative evidence based medicine', *Lancet*, vol. 371, pp. 296–7.

Frankel, R. (2004), 'Relationship-centered care and the patient-physician relationship', *Journal of General Internal Medicine*, vol. 19, pp. 1163–5

51. THREE KINDS OF REFLECTION

Bakhtin, M. (1986), *Speech Genres and Other Late Essays* (Houston TX, University of Texas).

Palazzolli, M., Boscolo, L., Cecchin, G. & Prata, G. (1980), 'Hypothesising-circularity-neutrality: three guidelines for the conductor of the session', *Family Process*, vol. 9, pp. 3–12.

Schon, D. (1987), *Educating the Reflective Practitioner* (San Francisco CA, Jossey-Bass).

Vygotsky, L. (1986), *Thought and Language* (Harvard MA, Massachusetts Institute of Technology Press).

52. BRIEF ENCOUNTER

Boehm, C. (2012), *Moral Origins: The Evolution of Virtue, Altruism and Shame* (New York NY, Basic Books).

Buss, D. (1993), *The Evolution of Desire: Strategies of Human Mating* (New York NY, Basic Books).

Dunbar, R., Barrett, L. & Lycett, J. (2005) *Evolutionary Psychology: A Beginner's Guide* (Oxford, One World Books).

ACKNOWLEDGEMENTS

....

While writing these pieces I nearly always received helpful comments from family, colleagues and friends. I particularly want to acknowledge the steadfast support of two editors, Dr Christopher Martyn and Dr Fiona Moss, my wife Rabbi Lee Wax, and the late Dr Brian Snowdon. This collection is dedicated in memory of Brian.

AUTHOR'S NOTE

....

Seventeen of these essays, listed below, are adapted from ones that appeared in the *Postgraduate Medical Journal*, published by the British Medical Journal. The originals can be accessed in their full online archive at http://pmj.bmj.com/content. For further permissions for these, contact bmj.permissions@bmj.com.

The remaining essays are adapted from *QJM* (formerly known as the *Quarterly Journal of Medicine*).

37. THE FACTS OF DEATH

38. CARE PATHWAYS

39. ON KINDNESS

40. CAPABLE BUT INSANE

41. ON THE RECORD

42. CLOSE READINGS

43. MEET YOUR MICROBIOME

44. OPIUM

45. MEDICINE AS POETRY

46. THE BREATHTAKINGLY SIMPLE FACTS OF LIFE

47. MONKEY BUSINESS

48. MEDICINE UNDER CAPITALISM

49. MEMORIES OF THE WORKHOUSE

50. TAKING RISKS SERIOUSLY

51. THREE KINDS OF REFLECTION

52. BRIEF ENCOUNTER

53. POWER AND POWERLESSNESS

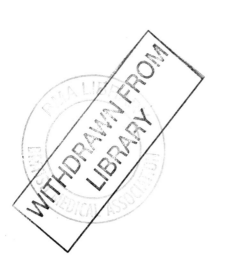